Adult Conductive Education

A practical guide

Melanie Brown
Ágnes Mikula-Tóth

Stanley Thornes (Publishers) Ltd

First published in 1997 by:
Stanley Thornes (Publishers) Ltd
Ellenborough House
Wellington Street
CHELTENHAM
GL50 1YW
United Kingdom

97 98 99 00 01 / 10 9 8 7 6 5 4 3 2 1

A catalogue record for this book is available from the British Library

ISBN 0-7487-3297-7

Typeset by WestKey Limited, Falmouth, Cornwall
Printed and bound in Great Britain by TJ International, Padstow, Cornwall

Contents

Acknowledgements

The authors would like to thank all the adult participants at the National Institute of Conductive Education in Birmingham for their support, co-operation and constant inspiration. Without them none of this would have been possible. They are the people behind this book and for whom it has been written.

The authors cannot write a book about conductive education without paying tribute to the Pető Institute in Hungary for all they taught us. They not only provided the knowledge base without which this book would not have been written, but provided services for large numbers of people from the United Kingdom. A special thank-you to Dr Mária Hári for her dedication to conductive education and for her excellent teaching to her students. A special thank-you also to the National Institute of Conductive Education, in particular to Andrew Sutton for providing the means for establishing this work within the United Kingdom and for their continuing desire to expand services and knowledge for the benefit of professionals, adults and children throughout the country.

A big thank-you to Dr Lillemor Jernqvist and Maureen Lilley for their invaluable comments and suggestions.

A special thank-you goes, too, to Pauline and Dudley Brown for their love, encouragement, understanding, support and belief that it would all be finished one day!

Introduction

This book has been written following a number of years of practical experience of conductive education with adults in the United Kingdom. During the 1990s there has been an increasing interest in this work from a number of professionals and it was felt that a practical guide was needed. Alongside this, there are a number of nation-wide training initiatives, from NVQ level up to degree courses, which will result in an increasing practice base throughout the country.

There is very little literature available on this subject and the theoretical background is still unclear. Despite this, conductive education is becoming an integral part of education and rehabilitation in the United Kingdom and, as such, more specific literature is required.

This book is not intended to search for a theoretical background to conductive education nor look at the subject only from a neurological point of view, but to provide professionals and participants with a working knowledge of the subject, complimented with any theoretical knowledge available. This book is designed to improve the practical, working knowledge of this area of expertise in order to provide quality services for adults with neurological conditions.

The book has been written from experience within the United Kingdom, and all practical examples are based within this culture. The knowledge base for this practice has, however, come from Hungary and been applied into the relevant context. Like any other educational system, conductive education has to work within the cultural background of the society and people to which it is providing a service.

Conductive education provides services for adults with a wide range of neurological conditions. This guide concentrates on the main conditions only; the underlying principles can be applied to a variety of conditions. Conductive education has very clear aims that can be applied in many situations and to many different conditions, but in order to do this the professional should have a good understanding of the underlying principles.

How to use the guide

This guide has been separated into three distinct sections, each one representing a specific aspect of conductive education in relation to adults with neurological conditions.

Part One should be read by both participants and professionals alike. It provides a working knowledge of conductive education in practice and forms the basis for the rest of the book.

Part Two covers the main neurological conditions gaining benefit from conductive education. Here, the reader may wish to focus on specific areas of interest, but should not be too drawn by diagnosis alone, since there will be some overlap between diagnoses.

Part Three includes a study of the participants' views on conductive education and a number of case studies. This section provides a valuable insight into the views of the service user.

This guide is not meant to be read from cover to cover. It is not a recipe for conductive education, but a guide to improve understanding of the system for both professionals and participants. At present there are still many mysteries surrounding this area of work and it is hoped that this guide will help to clarify these.

PART ONE

Roles Within Conductive Education

The conductor

1

This chapter aims to outline the background and training of the conductor as the professional who delivers conductive education. Included in this is a brief, general overview of specific elements within the role of the conductor, including:

- content and structure of training course
- the consultation
- conductive observation techniques
- programme planning
- facilitation
- the conductive group
- personality of the conductor.

This chapter should provide background information which will be expanded upon in subsequent chapters.

CONDUCTOR TRAINING

The conductor is the term given to the professional who delivers conductive education. This term, and indeed the profession itself, has been the cause of much discussion in Britain since the 1960s. As with every other profession, a conductor has to undergo some form of training in order to be able to use the title, for example, I would not call myself a teacher without a teaching qualification; the same is true of lawyers. We need, therefore, to look at the training of the conductor and where this knowledge base comes from.

Over the years there have been many varying reports of the substance of the training of the conductor, and this has resulted in misconceptions of the qualification. Naturally in an effort to explain to the British public, similarities were drawn with existing professions and existing systems. One school of thought is that the conductor is a teacher, nurse, physiotherapist and speech therapist all in one (Crompton, 1988; McKinlay, 1990).

In reality the conductor is a new profession, one that is not yet fully recognized within Britain. Stanley (1988) recognized this at an early stage, and, preceding this, The Foundation for Conductive Education sent 10 students to the Petö Institute in 1987 to undertake the four-year diploma course.

The conductor is a specialist in conductive education. Conductive education is:

> an integrated, complex education, a methodological planned and guided learning system, affecting and encompassing every single function of the child at any given age.
>
> (*Hári, 1990*)

In order to ensure that this definition is totally correct, the word *person* should be substituted for child, as conductive education is not limited to children but also includes adults with neurological disorders.

To be able to understand in more depth the knowledge base required for this specialist, we need to look into the syllabus and the training course. Fortunately this task is made easier by the fact that there is, at present, only one recognized training centre for this profession – the Petö Institute, Budapest. Many other shortened courses and familiarization courses are run throughout Britain and Europe, but there still, in 1996, remains only one centre where a diploma in conductive education can be attained.

CONDUCTOR DIPLOMA IN HUNGARY

Petö officially began his work in 1945 (Hári, 1990), and even at this time he was training his own staff even though this was not recognized. In 1963, the educational qualities of the system were recognized and the conductors became professionals in their own right in Hungary. In 1985, this was further expanded by close work with the Teacher Training College of Budapest, which led to a recognition of the conductor status in schools within Hungary.

In 1987, the Petö Institute saw its first intake of British students. Prior to this a small number of Japanese people had completed the course, but there had been a limited opportunity for foreign students. This opened up further opportunities for others and more foreign students attended, mainly from Britain and Israel.

In 1989, the International Petö Foundation (IPF) produced a document outlining the training course. This is the most recent available document and outlines the elements of the course. The following are extracts from this document.

The basic tasks of conductor training are to:

- prepare students for conductive education of the motor-disabled at every stage of life, providing sufficient professional knowledge and ability, as well as skills, in using them;
- provide the necessary knowledge, skills and competence to assess the dysfunctions, learn about and develop the personality and the community, work out an optimum conductive development programme and to plan and realize conductive education;
- raise the interest of students in sciences and self-education, develop the skill of innovative thinking necessary to perform conductive education and introduce the methods of research, development and experimenting related to the activities of the conductor.

PRINCIPLES OF TRAINING

These principles always relate to practical experience. The whole training course has a practical bias, the curriculum for training providing a link between theoretical and practical training. The topics covered are taught in larger groups, small groups and individually, in both practical and theoretical training:

> providing and improving knowledge, skills and expertise as well as the capacity to realize and identify problems and solve problems, which qualities are indispensable for entry into their profession.
>
> *(IPF, 1989)*

STRUCTURE OF TRAINING

The Hungarians run a two-term year, and the course consists of eight terms. Each term comprises 16 weeks with between 30 and 36 hours per week. Examinations are taken every year and a student must successfully complete one year before beginning the next. In addition to these annual examinations, the student has to write and defend a thesis as well as pass a state examination at the end of the fourth year. This state examination is both internally and externally monitored and has to comply with statutory regulations. If successful, the student will become a graduate conductor and is thus entitled to practise conductive education with people who have a motor disorder due to an impairment of the central nervous system.

CONTENT OF TRAINING

The content of the training as carried out in Hungary, amalgamates educational theory, the principles of conductive education and medical knowledge of neurological conditions. The following lists outline the areas of study over a four-year period.

- General studies
- Philosophy
- History of culture in education
- Ethics
- Physical education
- Foreign language (Hungarian for foreign students)
- History of Hungary.

Basic subjects relating to pedagogy, biology and psychology are:

- Education theory
- Teaching theory (logic)
- Education history (universal)
- General, developmental and educational psychology
- Psycho-diagnostic studies
- Functional anatomy, physiology, pathology
- Functional neuro-anatomy, physiology
- Paediatric studies, school health care
- Intrauterine development
- Infant neurology
- Neuropsychology
- Functional neuropathology
- Studies related to the improvement of the production of sounds and speech
- Methods of pedagogical research.

Complex and special subjects:

1. Symptom studies
2. Unit of subjects in general conductive education
3. Unit of subjects in special conductive education
4. Methods of rehabilitation
5. Conductive education of kindergarten age children
6. Education of language and hearing
7. General teaching of the mother tongue (reading, writing, grammar, speech)
8. Visual teaching
9. Music teaching
10. Nature and environment
11. Mathematics.

Subjects 5 to 11 are related to their role in the method of conductive education, and the methods of teaching the requirements, i.e. state requirements.

PRACTICAL TRAINING

A large part of the training is practically based. Throughout the eight terms the student will gain practical experience in large and small groups, and attend demonstrations and observational workshops. Practical examinations are also carried out each year; at first these are highly structured, but during the course the student will be required to become more independent. Success in annual practical and theoretical examinations is the criterion for continuing with training. In addition to the above, there are some elements of training which take place outside the set classes:

• orthotics, methods of neurosurgery, orthopaedics
• methods of preparing equipment
• education technique
• scientific research performed by students.

The International Pető Foundation states that the first two years of the training should be carried out in two languages, Hungarian and English, and from the third year only in Hungarian. In practice this is not entirely correct, as the student needs to be able to speak some Hungarian in order to communicate with the children and adults during their practical work. Although lectures are translated, there is rarely a translator available when the student is working in a group. There are some international groups for children and adults where English is the main spoken language, but these are few and far between.

As an English-speaking graduate conductor it is essential to have a working knowledge of Hungarian in order to establish a rapport with the people you are working with, and be able to ask questions and understand the practical application of the system within the daily work.

There are, at present, no British students at the Pető Institute. The last intake graduated in June 1993. In the period 1987–1993 a total of 15 students graduated, who had been sponsored by the Foundation for Conductive Education in Birmingham, and 10 graduated who had been sponsored by SCOPE (formerly the Spastics Society). The majority of graduate conductors working in Britain are still of Hungarian origin.

TRAINING AND THE FUTURE FOR BRITAIN

At the time of writing there are numerous schemes running which offer insight into conductive education, e.g. Hornsey Centre, SCOPE school for parents and The Scottish Centre for Children with Motor Impairment. There are in addition two schemes, one at Wolverhampton University and one at Keele University, for a full-time course leading to a degree (the British equivalent of a Hungarian Diploma) in conductive education. Keele University accepted their first intake of students in September 1996. There are also various schemes in progress to establish NVQ training.

In brief, the present training course is only available at the Petö Institute. This poses immediate problems as the qualification and professional status are not recognized in other countries. The system is spreading throughout Britain and there has been pressure from professionals for some formalized training. It is hoped that once a training course with a British qualification is established then the system will become less diverse and achieve acceptance among professionals in countries outside Hungary.

THE CONSULTATION

Conductive education, being a system of education, has to assess in order to determine whether the person will benefit from the system or not. Despite being heavily criticized for this (Bairstow, Cochrane and Rusk, 1991; McKinlay, 1990), and often seen as selection, it is no different from other forms of assessment we see in the western world. Adults with disabilities are constantly being assessed for types of equipment, services and treatment required, and so on. It is therefore vital that people are assessed for any form of specialist provision.

The term 'assessment' implies that the conductor is assessing whether the person is suitable for conductive education. The conductor is, in fact, firstly deciding whether conductive education is suitable for the person, and, secondly, they themselves are being given an opportunity to see whether conductive education is appropriate for their needs. In the light of this very important two-way process, the term **consultation** will be used in preference to assessment. This describes more the process that takes place once someone has applied for a place in the conductive education system.

Consultations will naturally vary according to the circumstances and place where they are being held, and it is impossible to include a blueprint for such consultations. There are strong guidelines and codes of behaviour to help the conductor discover how this system can help the individual concerned.

The following is a guideline based on a consultation carried out in Britain and, therefore, includes elements of information required for this society.

The aim of the consultation is for the conductor to find out what the person is capable of and not what they cannot do. This is the golden rule for the conductor. There are three key elements in the organization of the system of conductive education, as described by Hári (1984).

1. The careful grouping of the pupils, for the purpose of instruction, on the basis of several criteria.
2. The highly perfected team-work of the conductors and the conductors-in-training.
3. The nature of the interpersonal relations among the conductors themselves and those in their care.

For these reasons, the consultation plays an important role within the whole system.

APPLICATION FORM

If a person is interested in joining a group then it is usual for them to complete an application form. This enables the conductor to gain some background information about the person and prepare for their visit. An application form should include:

- name, address, NHS number, next of kin, date of birth
- medical diagnosis and date of diagnosis
- some detail of the present condition of the person with regard to their everyday activities, e.g. main method of moving around and equipment used, including wheelchairs, sticks or support; dressing skills; self-help skills and feeding skills
- general information on communication methods
- information regarding vision; particularly important if vision has been affected by the neurological problem
- relevant medical information; any history of heart problems, diabetes, epilepsy, serious medical conditions, or known allergies.

In addition, specific diagnostic information may be relevant, e.g. drugs taken, continence, contractures, etc. These are discussed in greater detail in the chapters on diagnosis in Part Two.

This information will give an overall picture on which the conductor will be able to base the consultation. It is very important that the consultation is tailored so that the conductor is able to start with the actual level of ability and then build on this.

The consultation could take place at the person's home or the centre they attend. The latter is usual because of resources and time. It must be stressed, however, that if the centre is the chosen venue, then the conductor must take into consideration that the person is in an alien environment and therefore may be very nervous and concerned that they will not be able to show everything they are capable of. The conductor must be empathetic to this and try to ensure that the person is as relaxed as possible.

FORMAT OF THE CONSULTATION

Firstly, the conductor must spend some time explaining the system of conductive education to the person; they must realize that it is not a treatment but a process of learning. It is often useful to liken this to a well-known example such as a slimming club. By attending a slimming club you will not lose weight; in order to lose weight you must take the information that you have learnt and build it into your everyday life. Once this happens you will begin to see results.

The group sessions within conductive education are learning sessions – the conductor teaches the person to learn (Hári, 1984). This is particularly true with adults who attend on a sessional basis. The learner then actively builds the skills learnt into their own lifestyle. They must play an active part in the process; they are not the passive recipients of conductive education. It is important that the person understands and is prepared to play this role, if not then it is possible that conductive education is not a suitable system for them. The conductor works with the person and does not 'do to them'. The person is not a recipient but an active participant.

Throughout the whole of this time the conductor will also have been observing the spontaneous movement of the person: their sitting position, ability to change position, communication level, level of concentration and their reactions in a spontaneous situation. This is the main part of the consultation for the conductor, as the information gained during this stage will be the information on which individual goals can be set. Spontaneous movement is the basis for any improvement and not the movements they are able to produce when requested. Spontaneous movement becomes learnt movement. It is from this baseline that the conductor will work with the person.

It is also important for the conductor to observe specific movements, e.g. changing position from standing to sitting to lying, rolling over, range of movement of limbs, hand–eye co-ordination. All these elements will be observed in a short movement session that is structured to include all the above elements.

The following is an example of a more structured observational session. Each consultation should be tailored for the individual concerned.

1. Ask the person to make their way to the plinth/bed by whatever means they are able.
    OBSERVE
    If able to walk:

    - weight bearing
    - transference of weight
    - posture
    - position of head, shoulders, trunk, hips, knees, feet
    - where the movement is initiated (i.e. from hips, shoulders, head)
    - length of step with both feet
    - flexing of knees, hips, ankles
    - balance
    - rhythm of stepping
    - symmetry of body.

If unable to walk:
- form of assistance required
- ability to control wheelchair
- co-ordination
- posture
- symmetry
- position of limbs and trunk.

2. Ask the patient to sit down on the bed and take shoes off.
OBSERVE

- ability to turn around
- balance when changing position
- gravitational point when sitting down (i.e. do they have control, do they flop down)
- symmetry
- balance in a sitting position
- flexing of hips
- ability to lean forwards and maintain balance
- fine motor control
- transference of weight when taking shoes off.

3. Ask the patient to lie down in centre of plinth/bed.
OBSERVE

- ability to transfer to lying position
- position of body
- symmetry
- awareness of body in space
- position of head, trunk, arms, legs, feet.

4. Ask the patient to lift legs up individually, bend legs, take legs apart, roll over on to one side then the other, sit up.
OBSERVE

- range of movements
- contractures
- painful movements (usually done by watching the person's eyes, as they often will not say)
- lateral co-ordination
- symmetry of right and left side of body
- whether the movement starts from the appropriate position (often head movements will be used to initiate difficult movements like lifting legs)
- use of hands
- movement of digits
- ability to produce isolated and combined movements.

5. Ask the patient to sit on edge of plinth/bed, stand up (if appropriate), lifting arms.
   OBSERVE

   - ability to weight-bear on legs
   - balance
   - range of movement of arms, hands, fingers.

   In addition to the above points, the conductor should also observe:

   - ability to understand instructions
   - perceptual abilities
   - relationship of body parts to each other and in space
   - tremor, range and type
   - overall co-ordination
   - confidence in abilities.

It is usual that the conductor will build on this basic example, according to the diagnosis and main problems. It may be necessary to ask the person to read or write something or use a cup. As this can only be appraised during a consultation, the conductor must be flexible and react to the individual situation.

Following this the conductor should ask what are the person's own, particular aims; what they would like to achieve and what they expect to achieve. The conductor must remain honest and realistic, and recognize the difference between dealing with a progressive or non-progressive condition. The conductor should also be able to tell the person immediately what short-term goals could be achieved through conductive education, and discuss these with them. Recommendations can be made for the type of provision required to meet these needs and the appropriate group (or individual session) for this.

If it is felt that conductive education would not be suitable, then the person should be told at this stage. In general, this situation would arise if, perhaps, the person has severe medical problems affecting their ability to actively participate. If there was doubt then the person would be offered a trial period, during which everyone concerned could determine whether a placement would be beneficial.

Finally, the person should receive a written copy of the consultation and be given the time to decide whether they wish to take up the recommendations. During the whole consultation the applicant should be a partner and able to make their own decisions about the goals and provision they would like. This partnership is essential, as the conductor is there only to guide the person through the learning process, not learn for them. If this is established at the beginning, then the person will feel confident and this will assist their future success.

CONDUCTIVE OBSERVATION

Observation does not end once the person has attended for consultation; it is ongoing. There are two very specific types of observation in conductive education.

OPERATIVE OBSERVATION

There the conductor is concerned with how the person carries out the task and what support is required to do this.

PROGRESSIVE OBSERVATION

The conductor is concerned with how the person solves the tasks and how the solution to the task is developing and changing. This observation focuses on the programme as a whole and not on the individual tasks. The conductor gains a detailed knowledge of the techniques the individual is using and this allows them to assist the person in applying these in other situations.

The conductor collates information from both these forms of observation and uses this to set or change the aims and solutions for the individual. Any situation, whether it is during the task series or a spontaneous situation, can be used for progressive observation, this then acts as a base for a higher level of learning.

PROGRAMME PLANNING

The programme in conductive education includes all the elements needed for the optimal level of activity for the group. When looking at the work with adults with neurological conditions, we are looking at a programme which lasts for approximately two hours. Unlike the work with children, adults attend on a sessional basis and for a part of the day. Since we are looking at a system of education, this session has to provide the basis and opportunities for the person to learn. The learning of an action is a cognitive process and the programme must be designed to enable this.

A neurological disorder affects the automatic, voluntary movements of the person. Some of the skilled movements that they have learnt through their life are no longer automatic, they need to be relearnt. In order to learn a skilled movement, each part must be carefully timed and executed in the correct order.

Example

If we are fortunate enough to be able to walk without thinking about it, then we have automated a sequence of skills. Most of us will not remember doing this as it happened, quite naturally, at a very early age. We no longer have to think about how to stand on our legs, how to transfer the weight on to one leg to allow us to step with the other one; we do not have to think about how we step and where we step; we do not have to try and find our balance point. In fact, if we miss any of these stages, or do not accurately perform them, then our body will automatically correct itself.

For the adult who has lost or is losing this skill, those parts of the movement which were automatic have to be made conscious. They have to be learnt again, sometimes in a different way.

The same is true of all our skills, whether they be buttoning our shirt, washing ourselves or drinking from a cup. The programme must include all those movements we use in our daily life. The way in which these are solved and the combination in which they are used is individual.

The programme aims to arm the person with the skills required to perform the activities that we take for granted. It is impossible to prescribe a solution to how to walk, how to write, how to hold the soap, how to get out of bed. If we observe human behaviour, we find that each person has their own individual solution to all of these skills, and the person with a neurological disorder is no different. We can teach a person the elements of a skill and the sequence and rhythm in which to perform them, but we cannot teach them how to solve it – this is the individual's own solution.

The programme must, therefore, contain the elements required to equip a person with the skills needed for their daily activities. There are only so many movements to make with the head, shoulders, trunk, wrists, knees, etc. These movements will be the same throughout all forms of rehabilitation. The conductor, however, has to plan the programme so that the person learns how to perform and use these movements in the most appropriate way for them.

The programme must be logical. The tasks need to build on each other; the success of the second one depending on the success of the first, and so on. If I want to put my hand on my head, I need to be able to bend my elbow, lift my arm and have the co-ordination to place my hand on my head. This sequence could be included in a task series. There must be logic to the movements and the person must be able to see the connection between tasks.

For the adult, it is usual for the programme to consist of the following elements:

- task series in a lying position
- task series in sitting position, using larger movements of upper body
- task series involving finer co-ordination
- a practical activity, perhaps a life skill or craft
- task series in sitting position, looking at posture and leg and trunk movements
- task series in standing position
- task series for walking (if appropriate).

These elements may be adapted for a specific group, but in general this format would be followed. The task series may be combined or more specific ones may be added, e.g. to work with facial expression and gesture.

The combination of the task series is the programme. The programme should be fluent with a smooth transition from one element to the next. The skills or techniques learnt in one task series should be used and practised in the next. The rhythm of the group is not only applicable to the task series but to the whole of the programme.

When planning the programme, the conductor needs to start with the level of the group, looking at the skills they have and how these can be built on. The task series must include the elements of the skills which the person will use and relate to the task, otherwise it becomes abstract. Once the task is concrete then the person is able to apply it to any situation they want to, whether it be pegging the clothes out or mowing the lawn.

Example

One position which is taught to ensure stability is to stand with hands on hips. For one person this may mean security when standing at the stove, for someone else it may help to give stability when casting a fishing line. The conductor cannot say which movements to use and when as this is the individual application of the system. Just as with any other learned skill, each person will apply them in a different way. This is very important, as it allows the individual to retain their own personality and their own traits. The conductor must be able to give guidance and suggestions, but it should be stressed that, despite this, it is not the aim of the conductor to teach functions but the components which lead to the person being able to function. These components constitute the programme.

FACILITATION

The *Oxford Dictionary* definition of the term facilitate is: 'make easy, promote an action or result'. Conductive facilitation is exactly this; it is the methods used to promote an action or a result; to make easier. The main facilitator is the conductor, it is their role to guide the person, not to perform the action for the person. Facilitation can take many forms. It may be educational facilitation, which includes motivation, direction and demonstration, or mechanical facilitation, such as use of gravity, manual and synergistic action and fixation.

The test of any facilitation is whether it can be removed. If it can be removed then it is promoting a result; if it cannot be removed then it is replacing a result. A facilitation used by the conductor will be used with the aim of removing it, changing it and encouraging the same result without it at a later stage. Facilitation is not constant, it will change as the aim changes and as the person learns how to perform the movement.

Facilitation must also be used bearing in mind that the person receiving it will not always be in the same situation, will not always have the conductor next to them. They must be shown various ways of performing each action and learn ways of performing these without help.

The conductor has many forms of facilitation to draw upon. Manual facilitation should be one of the last used or should have a specific purpose. For example we may want the person to experience a certain movement so that they have an image of the end product. In this instance, the conductor may provide maximum manual facilitation. This, however, is not teaching the person to perform the movement but enabling them to work towards it, and it should only be done when absolutely necessary and should not need to be continually repeated.

METHODS OF FACILITATION

Modification of a task

Example

The task is to put thumb and index finger together. The person has a strong intentional tremor, so while trying to perform the task, the tremor increases and they are unable to do it. The conductor can ask them to pick up a straw from the table, and diverting their attention to a different activity the movement can be produced.

Example

The task is to stretch knees while standing. The person has a parkinsonian posture and finds it almost impossible to stretch knees when standing. The conductor may ask the person to push their hips forward and their shoulders back. This will immediately produce the desired movement; the person has achieved success by performing the task in a modified way.

Simplifying tasks

The conductor can help with a part of the task.

Example

The task is to lift the arms above the head in a standing position. The person finds that when they lift their arms they lean forward and feel insecure. The conductor may help the person at the hips. This is not passive assistance since the person is actively completing the task.

To do this, the conductor must know the aim. If the aim here was to improve control of the hips, then the conductor may simplify the task by helping at the shoulder. It is important that the conductor does not give help directly at the part which is producing an active movement, but they can help by securing another part to enable movement to take place.

Making use of assistance by the person

Example

No one knows better how to help than the person themselves. Sometimes they find it easier to walk if they have a line to follow, if there is someone in front or at the side of them. The conductor may stand at the person's side and gradually move one step away. It is vital that the conductor uses the person's own solutions and builds on these.

Dividing the task into sensible parts

If the task is to roll on to the right side and the person is unable to do so then the conductor should break this down.

Example

From a supine position, swing right arm to the side, bend left leg up, take left arm across the body, push with left leg, put left hand flat by chest.

Here the person has been able to achieve the task by learning the stages needed to do it. For many adults with neurological disorders this is the strongest method of facilitation. The sequence of movements which is automatic to most of us may no longer be automatic for them. If the action is broken down into sequential stages, then they are often able to perform it.

Positional facilitation

If the person is unable to perform a task in one position, then try it in another.

Example

The task is to lift the knee up, in a sitting position, and then clasp it. If the person is unable to do it, then they can try in a supine position. Once they have achieved it here, then they can use this skill to learn in another position.

Example

The task is to stretch the elbow. If the person finds this very difficult, they can try in a lying position, and from here they can try by rolling on to their side.

The use of varying positions enables the person to achieve active success, and they then have a base from which to learn this movement in other situations.

Linking movements

Similar movements can be linked, helping to strengthen the feedback.

Example

The task is to bend the wrists and lift the palms up. This can be accompanied by the same movement of the feet.

Example

The task is to lift the leg up. This can be accompanied by lifting an arm up.

Setting a more complex task

It can often help a person to be asked to perform a complex movement. This is a characteristic of people with Parkinson's disease. It appears that the concentration on a simple movement can cause tremor or dyskinesia, whereas if the movement is incorporated into a more complex one then tremor and dyskinesia do not appear.

Example

The task is to pick up a pen. The conductor can ask the person to pick up the red pen and put it behind the blue one on the table. The person is concentrating on the sequence and commands and thus the movement is often more automatic.

Connecting rhythmical speech

This is the basis of rhythmical intention, a powerful facilitation for the conductor. It has already been mentioned that each group will have its own rhythm, and this is connected to speech. Rhythmical intention is discussed in greater detail in Chapters 4 and 5.

The conductor, therefore, has many forms of facilitation to draw upon. The appropriate form will be chosen by the conductor, and the golden rule is to always use the minimum facilitation required to perform any task or activity. Once the person becomes used to a form of facilitation it is very difficult to remove it, they must be shown that success can be achieved in many forms, since this will enhance learning.

THE CONDUCTIVE GROUP

Group work is a part of the system of conductive education, but this does not mean that group work equals conductive education. However, the influence of the group for adults with neurological disabilities is seen as an integral part of the whole system.

The conductive group has been observed many times and there are varying criteria quoted (Sutton, 1984; Hári, 1988 and Russell and Cotton, 1994). In practical terms, the numbers within a conductive group will depend on many factors, i.e. the size of the premises, the number of conductors, the needs of the participants. This must not detract from the importance of the group and its influence on the individual.

Leighton (1972) recognizes that society is a collection of groups and each individual will belong to a number of these. He goes on to say:

> Human beings can be understood only in relation to other human beings. What man thinks of himself is his judgement of the reactions of other men to him.

When looking at an individual with a neurological disorder, whether this be Parkinson's disease, multiple sclerosis, an acquired head injury or as a result of a stroke, the person's image of themselves will have changed. They are likely to have spent some time within a group of people who are in hospital or have a similar condition. They will have begun to see themselves in terms of their condition, and the skills they had may be slowly deteriorating or may have suddenly been taken away from them. When placing these people together in a group they will naturally begin to compare themselves. It is the conductor's role to ensure that the conductive group does not become a collection of people with difficulties, but a collection of active people who are able to support each other and gain success.

From the initial meeting the conductor will have observed the skills that the person has and not the ones they have lost, and the person will take **their** skills and personality to the group. The conductor must create the right environment for the group. People must be active in their own learning process, and the environment must be active to allow them the opportunity to use the skills they have learnt.

TYPE OF GROUP

By definition the group will be heterogeneous. It is possible that the group members will have the same diagnosis, but there will be many individual manifestations of this. We know that there is no prescription for the progression of Parkinson's disease or multiple sclerosis; we know that there will be differences in the damage caused by a head injury or a stroke; and we know that cerebral palsy is a blanket term for many different problems. In addition to this we are working with the whole person, each with their own individual personality.

To provide success, the conductor needs to make this group homogenous. Russell and Cotton (1994) see the creation or gelling of the group as the first and dominant goal in conductive education. This can take place by:

- the creation of a completely new group
- the addition of a new person to an existing group

The first, creating a new group, will be the most time consuming and present the greatest difficulties but, it is what many professionals in the United Kingdom will face. Once established, the group then has to have the flexibility to allow new members to become integrated.

CREATION OF A NEW GROUP

How do we put people together in a group? We probably do not know them very well at this point. We can start with diagnosis: on a general level, we can assume that this will provide a pattern, structure and some common elements. Thus I may be starting with, for example, the following groups:

- Parkinson's disease (PD)
- multiple sclerosis (MS)
- head injury (HI).

The conductor will have an idea of their abilities from the consultation, but then must decide how they should be grouped.

Hári (1988) says that the uniformity of a group does not depend on the level of performance. A successful conductive group does not require each person to be able to perform at the same level. The members of the group need to be able to see success, achieve success, and share in the success of others. It is important to have a range of abilities within the group. The conductor, should ensure that each individual in the group is able to perform at their own level while maintaining success. It is therefore up to the conductor to see that the group gels.

ADDITION OF PERSON TO EXISTING GROUP

We will assume that this group has already gelled and is able to work together. When a new person comes in, it is important that the group is flexible enough to assist the person to feel part of the group. The integration of the person is the conductor's responsibility, and, by guiding the group, ensure its collective responsibility. The person will have been placed into the most appropriate group not by their level of performance but by an assessment of their needs, and in turn the group will adapt to accommodate this.

Whether there is a new group being created or whether there is a change in membership, the conductor's role remains the same. There are four elements which are crucial to the successful working of a conductive group:

- the rhythm of the group
- the structure of the group, including the programme

- the organization of the group
- the decentralizing role of the conductor.

THE RHYTHM OF THE GROUP

Each group will have its own unique, optimal rhythm which will have been established by looking at the individual needs of each member. This rhythm will be ever changing; it is not a set rhythm. It will be dependent on the needs and the personalities within the group. The rhythm will allow each individual to complete the task set in the optimum way. The task may be broken down or built up to allow for individual levels, but the rhythm remains constant for the group. It is this rhythm which provides a cohesive force for the group and provides the basis for the group to achieve success. This rhythm is described in more detail in Chapter 5.

THE STRUCTURE OF THE GROUP

The structure of the group will be formed through the programme set. This programme will consist of various tasks and activities relevant to the group. The tasks which are appropriate for, perhaps, a group with MS, may not be appropriate for a different group with MS.

The building up of the tasks will vary for each group, as will the facilitation required to perform them. The conductor needs to know the group and be able to respond to each individual at any given time throughout the programme. Without this the programme will fail, the members will not achieve success and the aims will not be reached.

A base programme may be set for each group, but this will be adapted by the conductor on a daily basis. This adaptation will only be learnt by the conductor through experience and knowledge of the individuals, and will take time to develop. The group needs to have common elements to ensure that gelling takes place and in order to do this the conductor must provide a common task, a common goal and a common activity.

THE ORGANIZATION OF THE GROUP

Organization is an important skill for the conductor. The conductor wants to teach people how to organize their movements, and in order to do this they must be able to work within an organized environment. The conductor has to know if someone needs specific help, whether this be verbal, manual or physical – it is important that the conductor does not wait for the person to fail before offering help. The conductor must predict where the problems may occur and intercept before they happen.

The room should be organized, equipment should be at hand, people should know what is expected of them and how they will be able to achieve this. All these elements are a part of the preparatory work of the conductor.

DECENTRALIZING ROLE OF THE CONDUCTOR

The conductor naturally assumes a leadership role over the group. In some circumstances this is essential, but the conductor should also be able to pass this role on to others. Leadership, within any group, is ever changing, and the group members must be allowed the opportunity to take on this role in order to maintain their active participation. Whilst doing this, the conductor must also be able to retain the elements essential to preventing the breakdown of the group.

PERSONALITY OF THE CONDUCTOR

The conductor should:

- be forward looking
- create a good atmosphere
- establish a positive environment
- provide flexibility
- supply organization
- have a knowledge of people and their needs
- nurture the rhythm of the group
- offer leadership
- pass on the leadership
- structure appropriate programmes
- give suitable facilitation to members
- build a framework for the solution of tasks
- maintain the uniformity of groups
- set goals and aims for individuals and for whole groups.

One observer at the Petö Institute summarized the role of the conductor when she noted:

> The conductors do not specifically look at one part of the person, they look at the whole person and a way for that person's achieving what he had not been able to achieve before because of his disabilities.
>
> (*Hayward, 1985*)

The role of the participant

2

This chapter investigates the role of the participant within the whole system of conductive education. It is with this understanding that the participant will be able to play an active role in their own learning process. The conductor must ensure that the participant is also clear about the role they can play within the group and their own learning process. Time should be allowed to explain this to each individual.

LEARNING AND THE PARTICIPANT

In conductive education, as with any other educational system, there has to be a two-way process between teacher and learner. Without this the teacher is unable to teach and the learner unable to learn. This relationship between the conductor and the participant is thus vital for the system to be effective.

The participants themselves have a role to play within this process, in that their learning has to be active. We cannot learn how to play tennis by watching a video at home; we may be able to learn the rules and techniques required but we would still not be able to perform those skills – the same is true of motor skills. The participant wishes to learn how to perform motor skills, and the conductor has the expertise and knowledge to teach them.

POTENTIAL FOR LEARNING

We often hear that a person with neurological damage is unable to learn due to this damage. When participants attend sessions, one of the first things to be looked at is how they perform their movements. In many cases we will see years of bad habits, just as we ourselves form; but if we are able to learn bad habits then we are also able to learn good ones.

Every human being has a potential for learning, although this may slow down with age or may be halted due to habits formed or other difficulties, such as neurological damage, whether acquired, congenital or progressive. Learning starts at birth and will continue until death. The rate of learning will depend on numerous factors, but learning will still take place. In order to achieve this, the participant needs an environment conducive to learning as well as the information on which to base this learning.

This is the base from which the conductor is starting and one that needs to be explained to the participant. Unfortunately, and all to often, they have been told that they will not learn any more, that they have reached the end of their rehabilitation or that they will only get worse. The participants need reassurance that they still have the capacity to learn. It may be that they need to apply this in a different way, that movements which were automatic need to be learned, or that they need to learn new techniques to overcome problems they face as a result of the neurological damage.

MOTOR LEARNING

Learning usually takes place by a continual cycle of feedback and correction. Motor learning is often split into two areas:

- motor learning as the acquisition or modification of movements
- recovery of function, which refers to the re-acquisition of movement skills lost through injury.

When talking about rehabilitation we are referring to the second area above. We tend to separate this from motor learning within normal subjects. Shumway-Cook and Woollacott (1995) suggest this may be misleading and that the two forms of motor learning cannot be distinguished from each other. Following this line of thought, we are then faced with a number of theories of motor learning. It is not our intention in this book to look at these theories in detail, but each participant must understand that they are able to learn motor control and increase their level of skill, and that in order to achieve this they must play an active role within their own learning process.

Each participant who attends a conductive education session attends in order to learn how to perform motor skills. This brings a very stark distinction between therapies, treatment and education. The participant will not be **treated** by conductive education because it is not a treatment; it has no start and no finish; it has no prescription. Therapies tend to be a combination of treatment and movement practice. The participant may be active within a therapy session, may be learning movements, but they are not learning the **acquisition** of skilled movements. The movements they learn may be directly applicable to everyday situations, e.g. turning on the bed but if this is learnt as a **function** then the person will not be able to apply the rules of that movement to other situations.

The participant in conductive education learns elements of motor skills as opposed to functions. The conductor cannot teach someone how to stand up because each person will do it in a different way. We can teach someone the function of writing, but not teach them how to personalize this to become their signature. All our movements have a personal aspect, each one of us will perform them in a different way. The participant should not be awaiting a prescription for movement, but should learn how they perform the elements of movement. Once these have been learned then they can be applied to every situation.

Example

If a person learns how to lift their right leg off the floor, then they will have learnt an element of skill. This, in itself, is not a function nor is it a skill, but one element of many skilled movements. This, in conjunction with other elements of skill will enable the person to put their right sock on, get into the passenger side of the car, step with their right foot, get out of bed and so on.

Example

If, on the other hand, we teach someone to get out of bed, then we have to teach them in their own bed within their own environment if this function is to be useful. The movement itself will vary according to the circumstances in which it is performed. This may be very useful for the individual within their own home, but what happens if they go and stay with friends or relatives, go on holiday, into hospital or change their bed. It may be that they will not be able to perform this function in other situations unless they have been able to practise in many different beds.   .

This system is obviously not practical; we do not want to make people prisoners in their own home. Many of the participants we see have to stay in hotels during their visits to the Institute. One of the biggest areas of concern is that they are de-skilled while they are outside of their own environment. This is due, in part, to the fact that they have learnt functions and not how to perform skilled movements.

The rules of any movement must be learnt before they can be applied. The task series in conductive education teach the rules of movements and not functions. Once these have been used then the participant is able to apply them to the situation they are in and this increases confidence and independence. To increase dependence on pieces of furniture or certain environments does not increase the independence of the person but reduces it.

It is very important that the individual participant is clear about this learning process from the start. They must learn how to produce the movement, to register the feeling of a movement and the involvement of all parts of their body; only then will they be equipped with the knowledge to apply this movement to other situations – this is skilled movement.

GROUP LEARNING

Participants working in a group will automatically begin to compare their performance with others in the group. This can be beneficial because participants can learn from the experiences of others in their situation. It is very important, however, that they remember that they are not a clinical diagnosis but a **person** who has a neurological disorder. This means that they will never have performed functions in the same way as the person next to them, and that although their problems may be similar, their solution may be very different. The conductor needs to acknowledge this and help each individual to find the solution appropriate for them.

The diagnosis is not the most important factor; we need to look past this to the person, their personality and the best way of learning for them. The participant must also look past their diagnosis and direct their learning in a way that is suitable for them as a person. The techniques and advice a conductor may give should be applied to each participant and not to a whole group or for a diagnosis. The importance of this will be apparent in Part Two of this book.

AN ACTIVE LIFESTYLE

The participant has to take a lead in moving towards an active lifestyle. This does not mean that they are always moving around but that they have purpose and aims for the day.

Many ask if they need to practise the tasks at home. It is traditional, in western culture that if we want to be fit then we have to exercise. There is a fear that if we stop exercising we will lose the abilities we have. This is, in part, true, but not due to a lack of exercise. Any movement disorder will lead to an increasing problem with everyday activities; this in turn leads to a reduction in the number of movements performed, which leads to a loss in the ability to perform movements. If we exercise then we may be able to perform these movements, but we will lose them if we stop.

Human nature being as it is, unless we are totally dedicated there will come a time when we put off today what we can do tomorrow. To expect a person who finds movements difficult to exercise in a way that many of us would not follow is unrealistic. In addition this means that the diagnosis and the problems associated with it become the focus of the day.

The average person is awake for about 16 hours a day and movements can be used during this time, which is far more than any exercise regime. If movements are built into everyday life then they can be used throughout this time in a natural setting and with an aim and purpose. While specific activities or movements may be practised to assist with learning they should be used within a daily context to increase overall management of the condition.

The participants, therefore, must apply their learning from the sessions to their everyday life. One example of this would be to put the TV remote control away for an evening – by standing up from the chair, walking to the television, changing the channel, turning around, walking back to the chair and sitting down again a large proportion of the tasks covered by the task series have been applied to skilled, purposeful movements. This reduces the need to practise these tasks as exercises and gives the tasks a new meaning.

The participant, therefore, has an important role to play within the whole system. The conductor and the participant work together to find the most effective way of learning, each one bringing different skills to this process. The participant has as many skills as the conductor, but these may be in different areas. The combination of the two helps the participant to learn how to perform motor skills, thereby learning techniques which help with the management of their condition.

The crucial point is that learning does not stop; adults **can** learn and **do** learn daily. Motor skill is a specialized area of learning, one that most of us do not have to face but one which can be learnt at any level with specialized teaching. Just as a tennis professional will work with a specialized coach to improve their level of skill, a person with a neurological disorder resulting in a motor disorder may work with a conductor to improve their level of skill.

The role of the carer   3

This chapter aims to explore the nature and role of the prime carer, whether formal or informal, within the system of conductive education. Their varying roles will be discussed, together with how the conductor can assist carers alongside the participants. There will be a brief overview of the Community Care Act (1990), a discussion of the effect of neurological impairment on the family, and an examination of the role of the informal and professional carer in conductive education.

NATIONAL HEALTH AND COMMUNITY CARE ACT (1990)

To our knowledge, there is no literature available relating directly to the carer of a neurologically impaired adult and the system of conductive education. References are available to the role of the family with a motor-disordered child (Read, 1988; Haug, 1991) and there is some overlap, but invariably the role of parent and carer is different from the role of spouse and carer or sibling and carer.

Caring assumes a responsibility over and above the norms we expect between adults (Twigg and Atkin, 1994) and such relationships need adjusting accordingly. Carers cannot be seen in isolation from service provision as any form of intervention will have a direct effect on their role, which may take many forms, financial, providing transport, physical burden, and so on.

The implementation of the National Health and Community Care Act (1990) means that local authorities have a duty to provide all relevant information on services available, and thus there has been an increased awareness of the levels and types of formal/professional care available. On the other hand, there remains a forgotten section of the caring world. Hancock and Jarvis (1994) reported that there were 6.8 million people providing care for adults for more than 20 hours per week at the time of their study. All of these were unpaid, informal carers. Many were members of close family, but this may have extended into the close community.

In the light of this, it is important that the conductor considers both the formal and informal carer alongside the neurologically impaired adult. In addition, the guidelines resulting from the Community Care Act must also be reflected in the type and standard of service provided.

OVERVIEW

This Act clearly states as its aims:

- to enable people to live as normal a life as possible in their own homes or in a homely environment in the local community;
- to provide the right amount of care and support to help people achieve maximum possible independence and, by acquiring or re-acquiring basic living skills, help them to achieve their full potential;
- to give people a greater individual say in how they lead their lives and the services they need to help them to do so.

For the vast majority of professionals working in rehabilitation there is nothing new or revolutionary in these aims. These aims have been an integral part of their work in the past and will continue to be so into the future. Service users, however, through this Act, are in a position of empowerment. Any assessment should be needs-led and not service-led; this ensures that the needs of the person are catered for and not fitted into the service which provides for them in the neatest way.

In order to achieve this, local authorities are to 'buy-in' services from the private and voluntary sector. The transition to this model of working appears to be slow, but progress has been made. An example of this shows that an increasing number of adults with neurological impairments are attending conductive education sessions within the voluntary/private sector, and that fees for these services are being met by social services and health authorities. It is, however, generally accepted that a needs-led service requires infinite resources (Skidmore, 1994).

Historically, the services provided have been demand-led. In traditional systems there is a top-down thrust from management to the activities of the staff. The Community Care Act demands a bottom-up line where the consumer is the centre of the focus. This should lead to an increase in services which meet the needs of people and a discontinuation in those that do not. This appears to be the ideology behind the Act, but in practice this is harder to achieve due to the costs of and individual preferences for services.

According to Skidmore (1994) the 1990s would bring a shift in emphasis towards neighbourhood services. These will vary in size and in the number and range of professionals working within them. Despite the localization of provision, the informal carer will still remain the prime carer, and in some instances this may increase due to the enhanced ability for people to remain in their own home with supporting services.

There is a shift in the central focus of care, to some degree a return to a home-base. Because of this there would be an increase in the contact between professionals and informal carers, and despite back-up there are still fears on the part of the carers. Those who receive help in personal relationships will still struggle to obtain help from other sources to protect that relationship.

The situation has perhaps changed little since the onset of the Community Care Act. In 1983 Bayley (Brechin, Liddiard and Swain, 1983), writing about the cost of caring in terms of the physical strain, emotional stress and disruption of normal life, concludes that despite this, informal care still remains the true primary care. The picture 10 years on looks very similar.

Carers have recently been brought more into focus and two major developments have led to this: the rapidly increasing number of older people in our society; and care in the community, which largely suggests care by the community.

Caring can lead to isolation from your own community and/or, in some instances, your family. If we take into account the numbers of carers and acknowledge the service that they are providing, then we must involve them in the planning of services. To do this, Davidson and Hunter (1994) suggest four areas to be taken into consideration.

1. Recognition of the responsibility they have assumed and an acknow-ledgement that carers, too, will have needs. This should be built into the assessment process.
2. Information. Carers should have full information about services avail-able in their area and the benefits they are entitled to.
3. Practical help. This may take many forms and be regular or intermittent.
4. Emotional support. This again, recognizes that the carer is also a client with individual needs.

The professional working within this system, therefore has to ensure that the carer's needs are also met. This may be difficult, as it is impossible to assume that the needs of the carer and of the cared-for will be the same.

> Most carers do not want to stop caring, but the love and obligation they feel to the people they care for should no longer be an excuse for ignoring their needs.
>
> (*Davidson and Hunter 1994*)

EFFECT OF NEUROLOGICAL IMPAIRMENT ON THE FAMILY

Prior to examining the relationship between the informal carer and the conductor, it is essential to explore the position from which the informal carer is operating. The diagnosis of a neurological disease, such as Parkinson's disease or multiple sclerosis, or the effect of a traumatic injury, such as a stroke or head injury, will have an enormous impact on the whole family. It is quite common for the injured person to turn first to their family for emotional support. The family may be involved in trying to stimulate someone who is in a coma, and the result of this is that the family have a role to play that can be forgotten when assessing needs. The implications of the incident for the family are not always recognized in a way which would lead to help and support being provided.

Statistics show that between 40% and 50% of all marriages in which one partner has suffered a head injury ends in divorce (Senelick and Ryan, 1991). Caring for a person who has similar needs to yourself is easier. When these needs change or become more demanding, then the family member undertakes a change in role. This may have social, financial and emotional implications. Povey, Dowie and Prett (1981) cite an example where the person with the neurological impairment tends to feel guilty about the extra burden placed on their partner; in turn, the partner may feel annoyed and resentful because they have to forgo social activities.

The family members have a very important role in 'showing' the meaning of the disability for both the disabled person and the family as a whole. In order to do this they will need support and information. Unfortunately in these situations, human instinct often takes over and the carer feels that it is their role to care totally for their partner.

> There is sometimes an understandable tendency for the partner of an MS sufferer to molly-coddle the invalid. In many cases this has the unfortunate effect of reducing the degree of independence of the person with MS who becomes labelled as a patient incapable of carrying out normal household or occupational activities. This can lower the morale of the person and in certain ways lead to a deterioration in his or her physical condition.
>
> (*Povey, Dowie and Prett, 1981*)

This is not only true with multiple sclerosis but with any condition where the partner is afraid and unsure what to expect. If there has been a traumatic injury, the person is hospitalized and requires nursing for some time. It is then very difficult for the family to try to change their role gradually in line with the improvement of the person, which may sometimes be very slow and gradual. Thus the patient–nurse role remains as the model for the family to follow.

MODELS OF CARER

Twigg and Atkin (1994) identified four models of carer (Table 3.1). The role which the carer will adopt depends on the type of neurological impairment, the level of dependency of the person, the type of services provided and

Table 3.1 Models of carer

	Carers as resources	Carers as co-workers
Definition of carer	Very wide	Wide
Focus of interest	Disabled person	Disabled person with some instrumental recognition of the carer
Conflict of interest	Ignored	Partly recognized
Aim	Care maximization and minimization of substitution	Highest quality of care for the disabled person Well-being of carer as means to this

	Carers as co-clients	Superseded carer
Definition of carer	Narrow	Relatives
Focus of interest	Carer	Disabled person and carer, but separately
Conflict of interest	Recognized fully, but one way	Recognized, but in relation to both carer and disabled person
Aim	Well-being of carer.	Well-being of carer and independence for the disabled person, but seen as separate

the professional who delivers these. The expectations of the person they are caring for will also be influential. There are varying reports on the role of the informal carer and the role of the cared-for. These highlight the fact that each situation must be seen individually, as each will be unique and inevitably not fit neatly into a role model.

The following are extracts taken from various sources which highlight the possible conflicts between the carer and the cared-for. Help with daily living means that disabled people can be citizens in their own right, taking part in society and in personal relationships.

Carers' lives can be restricted because they share the limitations imposed on the life of the cared-for person. Caring involves a feeling of being responsible for the cared-for person.

(Twigg and Atkin, 1994)

Watching the person with MS doing jobs at an excruciatingly slow pace can be most frustrating for the onlooker as well as the individual.

(Povey, Dowie and Prett, 1981)

He looks like my husband but he's not . . . My husband's gone.

(Senelick and Ryan, 1991)

Few carers enjoy any real compensation for the heavy burden imposed on them and many, understandably feel resentful.

(Youngson, 1987)

I'd say we don't want to be cared for at all. I would say that we want to be facilitated, supported and empowered. Care to me has connotations of custody and of lack of control and of looking after somebody who is sick and getting basically worse . . . what I want is to have control over my life, but at the times when it's difficult to do that then I want the support to actually get through that particular time. I would say caring and care in the community is about control – maintaining us in a certain position – and it's about seeing disabled people as people with individual problems.

(Bornat et al., 1993)

In spite of the problems highlighted above, it is still, in general, felt that people would prefer to have helpers who have no qualifications and experience, and the majority of people still wish to live in their family environment. The families also wish to see their family member within the home and not cared for by professionals outside.

WORKING WITH YOUR LOVED ONE: THE ROLE OF THE INFORMAL CARER

In the light of the Community Care Act and the varying nature of the carer's role, the conductor, like all other professionals, needs to set and follow certain guidelines when working with both the neurologically impaired person (participant) and with the carer.

The first contact the conductor has will be during the initial consultation. It is vital that at this point the needs of both the prospective participant and their carer are assessed. This information will form the base upon which the conductor will build the working partnership. The consultation with the participant (discussed in Chapter 1) and the assessment of carers should be addressed simultaneously.

Conductive education clearly aims to help the person remain as active as possible within their everyday environment. Since it is an educational system it requires the active participation of the person, a partnership with the conductor.

The carer's role is more diverse. In many situations their role will be dependent on other services they receive, domestic help, respite care, financial assistance, support groups, medical advice, and so on. It will also depend on whether they have employment or other family commitments, the relationship they have with the participant and whether they live in the same house. There are as many forms of informal care as there are families attending for consultation. The conductor needs to acquire background information in relation to the above in order to provide a service which is inclusive of the carer and not exclusive.

It is very easy to assume that the carer wishes to play an active role, that they have the same commitment as the professional. In reality there may be a variety of roles which will become evident:

- playing an active part in the rehabilitation process
- supporting the active role the participant wishes to take in their own rehabilitation
- spending time pursuing their own interests and/or meeting their own needs.

The conductor must discuss and respect the wishes of the carer and build a programme for the participant that is realistic within these joint roles.

CARER AS CO-WORKER AND SUPERSEDED CARER

If we return to the models of care identified by Twigg and Atkin (1994), then the conductor is able to work with the carer as a co-worker and a superseded carer. Conductive education as a system of rehabilitation is unable to offer help to the carer as a co-client or as a resource, and the conductor may need to give information to the carer about where they could receive that kind of support.

In the majority of cases the carers want to help their loved one but are unsure of how to do this. Very often discussion of how the participant can play an active role in everyday tasks, with guidance and facilitation, is a relief to both the carer and the participant. It creates a positive atmosphere where the participant is able to achieve the things they are capable of, and the carer no longer feels the burden of having to do things for them. This way of working can be translated into the role of superseded carer. The needs of both sides can be met while working towards the independence of the person concerned.

On the other hand, it may be more suitable to provide a service for the participant leading to the same goals as in the above example, while the carer uses this time to meet their own needs of well-being. This model – the carer as a co-worker – tends to occur in situations where the level of physical care is demanding, or where there are additional behavioural problems caused by the neurological impairment.

PLANNING A PROGRAMME

The daily routine at home is a very important factor when a conductor is planning. As the Multiple Sclerosis Society point out (1990): 'Care could be enhanced if people are given a chance to explain their home routine.'

The conductor may work with the participant on a sessional basis, usually once or twice a week for one and a half to two hours, or they may work on a short-term fixed placement of one and a half to two hours a day, five days a week for a period of three weeks. It does not even require a calculation to see how small a percentage of daily life this covers. Since the conductor aims to teach the person the skills which will have an effect on their daily activities, the established daily routine is vital for progress. No system of intervention will have an impact when it covers such a small percentage of the person's life.

Before any planning takes place the conductor needs to know the role of the carer and have an outline of the daily routine of both the carer and the participant. Having established this, together with the aims for the participant, a programme can be established. This programme may integrate with others and the participants form a group, or an individual session may be preferred.

Present experience indicates that the role the carer will play within the sessions will depend on their level of responsibility, in addition to their role as carer and the level of physical burden they experience.

CARERS IN CONDUCTIVE EDUCATION

- **The carer with additional responsibilities**
  This person may fully support the participant but rarely plays an active part in the sessions. Other responsibilities usually involve small children, employment, or elderly parents. It is useful if they are able to attend on a periodic basis in order to follow progress. They would also attend for assessment and reviews. There may be additional contact either in person or by telephone.
- **The carer who supports and pursues their own interests**
  Usually this person will bring the participant to the sessions and then spend the time meeting their own needs. This may be shopping, visiting friends or spending time alone. If their partner is a member of a group, then very often an informal carers group also emerges. They may discuss their difficulties, form friendships and share interests. On their return, following the session, the carer is often a little more refreshed and actively shares information on the content of the session, the progress of their partner, etc. They will be involved in assessments and reviews and will, on occasions, stay to observe the session.

- **The carer who attends the sessions alongside their partner**
  This person will either observe the sessions, actively take part, i.e. perform tasks alongside their partner, and/or wish to learn how to facilitate their partner to continue this at home. They may attend all sessions, they will be involved in assessments and reviews; and the conductor will work with them to teach them how to facilitate, give advice on the application of skills learnt into everyday situations and discuss difficulties and problems which may arise.

All three roles are very important to both parties. Whilst considering the needs of the carer to pursue their own interests, we must not forget that the participant may also wish to do this and work alone at times. If there is a conflict of interests, then the conductor must act as a mediator and help establish a provision which meets all needs.

Any form of neurological impairment affects the individual's ability to perform tasks. This may mean that they need to re-acquire or relearn certain skills or learn new skills. Following this, it is the transfer of these skills into everyday activities that shows whether the learning has been successful or not.

It is in this role that the prime carer plays the greatest part. The conductor should explain carefully the aims of the work to the carer and set certain goals which they can play an active part in helping to achieve. The balance between this and the support given to the carer is vital to the success of the participant.

THE ROLE OF THE PROFESSIONAL CARER

The main professional who delivers conductive education is the conductor, but this is not to the exclusion of others who are significant within the daily life of the participant. For some this may be a professional carer or a team of carers. In order to enable the participant to practise skills learnt and apply them to their individual situation, it is important that all professionals involved are working towards the same goals. For this reason, having gained the participant's permission, the conductor should work with, discuss and help the professional carer.

This relationship may cause a conflict of interests. By definition the professional carer is employed to do the things that the disabled person is unable to do on their own. On the other hand, the conductor is employed to guide and facilitate the movements of the person to enable them to play an active part in all activities. A practical example is in dressing: the carer may dress the person; the conductor would teach the person how to dress themselves with minimal help.

It is important, however, to note that the two professions in fact complement each other, and do not in any way work against each other. There will always be certain things that the carer will have to help with, but by working closely with the conductor the amount of physical help can decrease and a new role may emerge – that of the enabler.

CONTINUITY

Continuity within the life of the disabled person is vital. They need to be able to feel in control of their own destiny; by encouraging them to play an active part in everyday activities, self-confidence, self-respect and motivation improve. The conductor alone is unable to have this kind of impact as they only see the person within the confines of the centre. The carer, on the other hand, knows the daily routine of the person, knows their home environment and is, therefore, able to help the conductor to set realistic aims for the person.

There are certain problems which may occur:

- the time factor; the carer may not have the time, due to their workload, to help the person actively take part, as this is often slower than doing it for them
- the carer may not have the confidence to try the things they have seen at the centre.
- the equipment required may not be available.

Most of these problems can be overcome with discussion. A realistic number of tasks can be set up which can be achieved within the time allocated for the carer. The carer can work closely with the participant at the centre, under the supervision of the conductor, and equipment can be adapted or substituted for the purposes.

It is vital, therefore, that there is close communication between the participant, the conductor and the carer. When the links in this chain break down, then the application of skills is affected, and this will lead to a loss in motivation and self-confidence.

The conductor alone cannot influence the daily routine of the person or the achievement of aims. In some instances the carer's role may be a supervisory, encouraging role to motivate the person to continue working towards their goals. In other cases it means actually facilitating the person to help achieve these. The carer may have to provide the situation within which the person can use their skills. This may mean a change in the role of the carer, but there is no doubt that they will still be fulfilling a professional role.

In practical terms, there needs to be close liaison between the carer and the conductor. It is quite common that more than one carer is involved. In this situation it is important that either one carer takes the role of prime carer and shows the others, or that all carers visit the centre on a rotational basis.

It helps if the aims, facilitation and needs of the person can also be written. We are all by nature quite lazy and will always find the easy way around something. People with neurological disorders are no different, they too may have a bad day and need someone to do something for them instead of struggling. They may also be depressed and need the motivation to use the skills that they have. The carer must be aware of this and react to the daily situation.

For this reason it is vital that meetings and discussions do not take place between professionals in the absence of the participant. They must be able to say what kind of help they require and when, and this will be ever changing. They should however never be denied an opportunity to learn and to apply the skills which they have; they should never be rushed and should be given the help to achieve success; they should never be criticized for any effort made, whether this produces the required result or not. The minimum help should be given to allow the person to achieve their aims and retain their self-respect. In some instances, a structured planning of each step of the activity allows the participant to play a greater role.

SUMMARY

This chapter has outlined the role of both the informal and the formal carers within conductive education. Just as it is important that the conductor creates an individual set of aims for each person attending, whether this be in groups or alone, it is also important that each carer is given this same respect.

Carers, in the main informal ones, play an enormous role in the lives of people with neurological impairments and this is becoming increasingly recognized by local authorities and professionals. The carer cannot replace the professional and, equally, the professional cannot expect the carer to continue with their work. Often the carer wishes to play an active role but needs the guidance and help from the professional in order to do this. The professional must work in co-operation with the carers to assist the achievement of set aims with the neurologically impaired person.

Conductive education as a system aims to help the person in their daily activities, and the carer must be a partner in creating and achieving these aims while still retaining the individual needs of the person concerned. It is important that the conductor does not work with the carer directly, but indirectly through the participant. The needs and wishes of the participant must remain foremost in all situations.

The role of language

4

This chapter explores the possible combinations of the English language that can be used within the task series. Each one will play an important role, and the conductor should be aware of how their own language can assist in the learning process for the individual participant. Intention and how it is used within the task series is also discussed here.

LANGUAGE AND THE TASK SERIES

The task series is one of the main elements of the system of conductive education. In general, adults attend sessions which last for one and a half to two hours. This session consists of a number of task series compiled as a programme to meet the needs of the group. The base for the task series is discussed in Chapter 12; this chapter outlines how these tasks should be presented to the participants. Terms such as 'chanting' often cause confusion for the professional delivering the service.

INTENTION AND FORMAT

In conductive education we actively encourage our participants to repeat the task before beginning it. This enables them to concentrate on the task at hand, assists with breathing, with preparation, and allows them to focus their movements. The verbal aspect of the task series is often referred to as intention. Intention is the will to act, it is a conscious decision involving the highest structures within the brain. It is a distinctive ability in humans, but people with a neurological condition are often unable to intend their actions in the same way as you or I. This does not mean that they do not know what to do or that they lack the will, but it means that they are unable to break down the elements of the whole intention and this leads to a difference between intended action and actual performance.

The tasks allow us to teach the elements necessary to produce skilled movements, the stages required, the involvement of the whole body. For most of us this is automatic, and for many of the participants it was at one time automatic but they now need to make this conscious.

Task series do not involve 'chanting' or repeating instructions. The conductor will always give the task in the 'I' form. This enables the movements to be personalized for each individual and helps the conductor to guide the individual.

One of the biggest problems is when to use this format and when it is not required. All too often we hear people saying, 'I lift my cup up', while having a cup of tea. The verbal intention is only required within the task series, it does not mean that the individual needs to verbalize all their actions. It is a learning tool and not a method of achieving movement. If we restrict this learning tool to the task series then we must be very clear about the language used to achieve this. Adolescents and adults often find it very unnatural and sometimes embarrassing to verbalize their actions.

PLANNING THE LANGUAGE

The easiest way to plan the language used within the programme is firstly to ask ourselves how we would feel. Are we quite happy to be saying 'up – up' or 'down – down'? How do **we** use speech to regulate our own actions? In what format? Answering these questions will give the first insight into the language required for the programme. The language in children's groups should be quite different from the language in adult groups because of the different needs. Equally the language used in a group with aphasia should be very different from that used in a group with Parkinson's disease.

There is a tradition in the United Kingdom to use task series which have been translated from Hungarian. This is quite natural since Hungarian is the mother tongue in conductive education. When doing this, however, we should be aware of any differences in the use of language and not confuse this with the use of verbal intention. The conductor must be very clear in their usage of language and if in doubt should consult with a speech and language therapist.

There are many ways of saying each task and the conductor must choose the format which is the most appropriate for the group.

Each one of these will produce the movement required for the task. The task, however, does not consist only of a movement but must contain all other aspects relevant to skill development. In Hungarian there are fewer ways of saying the same thing and grammatically only one correct form. In English we do not have the benefits of this.

If the verbal intention is too long then it is possible that the participants

---

Example

The task is to bend the right knee and put the foot flat on the plinth while in a supine position. Any of the following could be said to achieve this:

- I bend my right knee and put my right foot flat
- I put my right foot flat
- Put right foot flat
- Right foot flat.

---

will lose concentration, become bored or feel self-conscious. The language content must also have meaning and be appropriate to the needs of the group.

If the group members have Parkinson's disease, and one of their main problems is the initiation of movement, then the conductor will not want a long gap between the intention and the action. This is the gap the conductor is trying to teach them to close, so they need a short intention, e.g. Right foot flat. If, on the other hand, the group members had severe spasticity and needed time to prepare for a movement, then the conductor would use a longer intention, e.g. I bend my right knee and put my right foot flat, or, I put my right foot flat.

If some of the group members had receptive aphasia, the conductor would not use an intention that was too complex for them to understand and/or repeat. In this instance they may initially say, Right foot flat, and then gradually increase this to, I put my right foot flat. The same may be true of those with expressive aphasia.

It is possible that the conductor might say, 'I put my right foot flat', but that members of the group would only say, 'foot', 'flat', or 'right'. This would depend not only on their movement abilities but on their language skills. For some it is appropriate for them to say the intention quietly to themselves at first. This is particularly true when we examine the concentration and effort required to move and speak, a skill which we would teach the participant since isolated movements cannot be used in everyday situations. We may need to gradually build up to achieving this.

The language used in the task series plays a very important role in the total learning environment. In English it is common to use the imperative form when talking to ourselves, e.g. Put right foot flat, Go shopping, Stand up, etc. In Hungarian, this form would not be used since it is not considered respectful to the individual. The imperative can be used very successfully with people suffering from Parkinson's disease as it helps them to initiate the movement. For English speakers, the imperative is not seen as inappropriate providing the appropriate intonation is used.

INTONATION AND FEEDBACK

Intonation also plays an important role in the task series. Through intonation the conductor can help the individual to prepare for a movement. If this preparation involves relaxing the body before initiating movement, then the intonation has to depict this, if it involves speeding the movement up, then intonation can be used for this.

The following examples show how intonation can be used in the task series to assist the overall aim and to maintain the flow of the movements.

Example

I put my right foot flat.

Here the stress may be on the word I as this is important, the rest of the sentence has a constant intonation. The emphasis can be placed on any key word, e.g. foot, right, or flat. This will depend on the nature of the problem.

I put my right foot flat.

Here the emphasis may still be on the I, but the intonation leads up towards the action. This will produce an immediate movement and reduce the time between preparation and action.

The conductor can use the voice in many ways to assist in achieving success. The presentation of the task series is very important as is the flow between tasks. Tasks within the task series are built on each other and the conductor can use intonation to link these. There should not be a long gap between tasks as this will prevent the movements from building on each other.

The conductor also uses language as feedback for the participant within the group. If a participant has performed a movement then they must receive feedback on how they have done it. It is very important to remember that adults need and enjoy praise as much as children. Language should be carefully used to be appropriate for the adult, to provide the best medium for achieving the aims set and the necessary feedback to improve performance.

It is not the aim that the participant will only be able to produce a movement if they have first said it to themselves; the aim is the opposite. By breaking down the neurological process in skilled movements we can correct them and teach the participant to perform movements consciously and in a skilled manner. Situations outside the structured programme can be used to implement this, such as coffee time. At this time we do not expect the participant to say what they are going to do or talk themselves through it out loud, but they may find it useful to use this technique in order to gain some control over their movements. Participants suffering from Parkinson's disease, however, often find that verbalizing the movement assists them in initiating it and as such enhances the ability to perform skilled movements.

In addition to language in the tasks, we also use rhythm to assist with the movement. This is discussed in detail in the next chapter.

The role of rhythm

5

This chapter examines skilled movement in relation to rhythm and looks in detail at the ways of using rhythm in conductive education. It should be read in conjunction with the previous chapter to gain an understanding of the concept of Rhythmical Intention as used in conductive education.

RHYTHM AND MOTOR SKILL

All our movements are rhythmical, and each part of a movement has to work in an appropriate rhythm if the movement is to be skilled. We can produce movements in isolation but if these are not connected in the correct rhythm then our overall movement will not be skilled.

KINETIC MELODY

Let us take the example of writing.

We may be able to write all the letters separately and neatly, but if we cannot join them together then we will not be able to write fluently. Once this has been learnt, it can be performed automatically and it becomes very difficult to stop in the middle of a word, or pick up in the middle of a word. The signature becomes one movement and not a series of movements. This is referred to as **kinetic melody**, a concept introduced by Luria (1973); it shows that as this process develops we are no longer dependent on the stages but on the whole, which becomes one single 'melody'. This involves a change in cerebral organization.

Neurological damage affects this kinetic melody and the stages involved in the activity become a series of single acts, each requiring a separate impulse from the brain. This means that the signature is no longer one movement, but that each letter formation has to be produced separately. The rhythm of the movement as a whole has been broken down, there is no flow between the parts, no connection between the separate elements.

How many times do we hear people say that they have to think about each stage of their movement, or that they have to think before they move?

Thus skilled movement is dependent on an overall rhythm, a rhythm for the whole and not a series of parts. The whole action is produced with one impulse rather than a series of smaller impulses. Movements which are automatic rely on this single impulse. We are able to stand up from the chair without thinking about transferring our weight, sliding forward, putting feet on the floor, etc. For the person with neurological damage this may not be so.

RHYTHMICAL INTENTION

Rhythm therefore becomes not only a powerful tool but the means of achieving skilled movement. This is why we hear the term **rhythmical intention** in conductive education. The task becomes the **intention,** the time given to perform this, the **rhythm.** The individual learns how to perform the movement and is then able to use this to increase the overall level of skill. If they have learnt the parts of a movement, such as getting into the car, then these can be sequenced together. Once this is done, a new neurological structure will be formed which means that they only need to intend getting into the car and the rest of the sequence will follow, i.e. the kinetic melody will have been formed.

The task series enables us to teach the sequence of a movement, the components and the order, but it must also allow us to teach the intention as a whole, so that our signature, for example, becomes the intention and not the individual letters of our name; standing up becomes the intention and not the sequence of movements required to do this. The person should be able to produce the movement or skill required without having to initiate each part of it. For this reason, each task in the task series is a complete movement.

In the last chapter we used the task of putting the right foot flat. If we follow this through, we now need to look at the rhythm required to enable this action to become smooth and skilled and not a series of smaller actions.

- The first stage has to be that the sequence of the movement must be correct. This should be broken down by the conductor: before beginning the movement, relax; transfer weight slightly on to left side to allow right leg to bend; lift knee and at the same time slide heel back (toes need to be lifted slightly to allow heel to move); head and arms should not be involved, hip should remain on the plinth, etc. There may be a problem in any one of these elements, and the conductor can use the task to assist in correcting this.
- Next we give the rhythm in which to perform the movement. This will allow the movement to be performed as a whole and give the melody

between the parts. This rhythm is usually given by counting but other media can be used if appropriate. We will use counting as the main medium for giving the rhythm to produce the skilled movement.

In the task series we usually count from one to five. The main reason for this is that it is an automatic sequence for most of us. This reduces the need for the individual to concentrate on the counting and allows them to use the rhythm more effectively. If, however, the person needs to learn or relearn this automatism, then the task series can also provide the medium for doing this in an active way.

The whole task would be:

I put my right foot flat 1 - 2 - 3 - 4 - 5.

- There should not be a break between the verbal intention and the rhythm for performing the movement. The person should begin the movement on the count of one, the verbal intention allows them time to prepare for this. The conductor needs to use intonation to ensure that this becomes a whole. The rhythm of the verbal intention should depict the rhythm of the counting, this again gives the person time to prepare for the pace of the movement.

The rhythm given will depend on the extent and nature of the neurological damage. As already described we may have to break the whole movement into parts and give a rhythm for each part. On the other hand, it may be possible to look at the whole movement and give an overall rhythm. This refers to the use of facilitation, and the reader should refer to the section, Facilitation, in Chapter 1 for details on methods of facilitation.

TEMPO, PACE AND INTONATION

The tempo, pace and intonation used have to be appropriate for the group, and they will differ according to the group and their main symptoms. As with the language used in the task series, the intonation is very important.

A person suffering from Parkinson's disease will need to learn to produce the movement on the count of one, as this allows them to initiate their movements in an appropriate and useful manner. This applies also to someone with dyskinesia or over-movements. Since over-movements increase in amplitude over time, they will begin to lose control over their movement. For this group, the movement should not be sudden, but direct, whereas the person suffering from Parkinson's disease will need the movement to crescendo on the count of one.

The person with spasticity should learn to perform the movement in a slow, relaxed way, to prevent the spasticity from increasing and to allow time to learn how to move without inducing spasticity. Therefore the intonation should be constant and not build up to the count of one.

A distinction has to be drawn between tempo and speed. Those who need to produce a direct movement, such as people with athetosis, dyskinesia or Parkinson's disease, do not have to produce a quick movement. The rhythm used to assist them will not necessarily be quicker than the rhythm used for those with spasticity, but they will need to produce a direct movement. The tempo of the rhythm can be the same for the whole group, where some take the full count to perform the movement and others perform the movement on the count of one and maintain it for the rest of the count.

Whilst the connection between the task and the counting is very important, it is also important to ensure that the whole of the count, until five, provides the intonation and rhythm required. The movement should finish on five, and our intonation should show this. We should not raise our voice to finish on five but drop it slightly to mark the end.

It is also possible that we will want to teach the rhythm between a sequence of movements, and for this we may perform a separate movement on each count.

Example

Arms to the side	1
Clap above head	2
Arms to the side	3
Clap to the right	4
Arms apart	5
Clap to the left	6
Arms apart	7
Hands down	8

Here the conductor is teaching the person how to sequence a series of movements in the appropriate rhythm.

GROUP RHYTHMS

It is impossible to give the rhythm for each group since each group will vary according to the task and its individual members. As with music therapy, the conductor needs to start with the rhythm of the group and then gradually influence this. A conductor cannot impose a rhythm on the group, but must assess the rhythm of the group and use this as a starting point. This is a skill which takes many years to acquire and can only come through practice. If the group loses the rhythm, then it is likely that the conductor has not found the appropriate rhythm and should change it accordingly. The conductor's own rhythm will be different from that of the group and they should be sensitive to this.

It will not always be possible to find the appropriate rhythm for each member of the group all of the time. The conductor therefore needs to adapt the rhythm used during the programme and use other methods of facilitation to ensure that everyone in the group is working at their own level.

Rhythmical intention is one of the main tools of conductive education, and used successfully it can ensure an increase in control of movements, in level of skill and in the automatism of activities. Participants can use this technique in any situation – it is completely portable and only needs to be used until the kinetic melody is formed. Once this has been formed the movement will become automatic.

In some conditions, such as Parkinson's disease, the use of rhythmical intention increases as the condition deteriorates. In this instance it can make the difference between the ability to perform actions or not. The power of this should not be underestimated by either the conductor or the participant – it is the most effective tool we possess.

The role of equipment 6

The use of aids and equipment in conductive education is considered in this chapter. It will include the use of aids available within the United Kingdom as well as the traditional wooden furniture often associated with this system.

TRADITIONAL FURNITURE

One of the first things that comes to notice when a visitor goes into groups at the Petö Institute is the furniture, so much so that it has become a feature of schools and centres around the United Kingdom. Many people believed that conductive education could only be 'done' with this furniture. We know now, of course, that this is not the case. An educational system will use its tools for learning, but this is all that the furniture represents. It would be impossible to expect every household to have this furniture and would detract from the essence of the system.

SLATTED BED/PLINTH

This furniture is, however, an increasingly common sight around the country. It has a very functional purpose. Figure 6.1 shows the traditional slatted bed, or plinth, which is regularly used. The slats enable the person to hold on to the bed when performing certain tasks, which helps them to learn how to fix their limbs and also provides security.

It is also very hard and can be uncomfortable. If this is so, then appropriate mats should be used on the plinth. It is a sturdy piece of equipment and thus provides stability. It is appropriate for people of varying height and weight and is useful in a centre where there are a number of groups attending. It can also have a wooden top placed on it which allows it to be used as a table. However, this is not usually appropriate for adults as it is often too low for them to sit at comfortably.

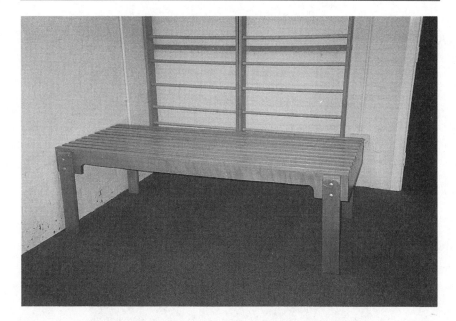

Fig. 6.1 Slatted bed/plinth

The plinth has a functional use and the effectiveness of conductive education does not depend on the furniture being correct. A divan bed with a firm mattress can also be used successfully as a teaching medium.

LADDER-BACK CHAIR

The ladder-back chair (Figure 6.2) is another common piece of furniture. Again, this has a good functional purpose in a centre where there are a number of people of varying height. It enables the person to hold a rung which is at a suitable level for them and adjust the position of their hands according to the task.

This chair can be used for any task in a sitting or standing position. If the individual is going to sit on it, then care must be taken that the seat is at the right height to allow the person to place their feet on the floor for security. It should also be borne in mind that sitting on this chair for any length of time is very uncomfortable, so other chairs should also be available for the person to use.

Wooden furniture retains the cold and in winter can be very cold to sit on. If this happens, then an appropriate covering should be put on the seat. When a person is learning to stand up holding on to the chair the conductor should not support the seat of the chair or sit on it. If the chair is completely stabilized by someone sitting on it, the person will have no feedback from their movements and will be unable to learn how to transfer from sitting to standing.

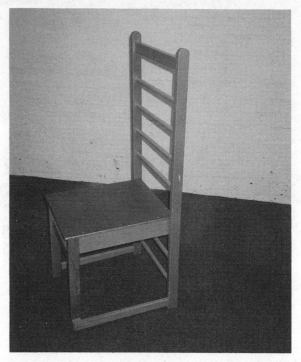

Fig. 6.2 Ladder-back chair

SLATTED STOOL

Slatted stools are also seen in the conductive education setting. They enable the person to sit on a stool without support and help to teach correct posture. Figure 6.3 shows a traditional slatted stool. The slats allow the person to hold on to the chair if necessary for added security. Sitting on a stool is very useful but can also be achieved on a household stool.

FOOT BOXES

Figure 6.4 shows the foot boxes which are often used. There is no mystery about their use. They are used if the chair is too high to allow the person to place their feet on the floor, usually young children rather than adults. Therefore those working with adults would not often make use of this piece of furniture.

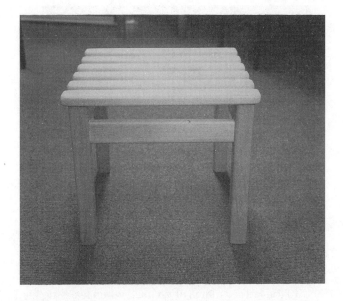

Fig. 6.3 Slatted stool

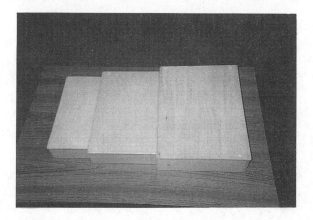

Fig. 6.4 Foot boxes

BATONS

Figure 6.5 shows two main types of baton that may be used in a task series. These pieces of equipment are useful for teaching symmetry, grasp and release. They may also be used when walking to help maintain balance by keeping the arms in an appropriate position.

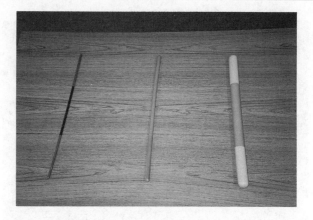

Fig. 6.5 Batons

LADDER

Figure 6.6 shows the ladder that is often used when teaching walking. This is a very useful piece of equipment as it provides a physical aid to help the person learn the symmetry of stepping. It is very important that the rungs are placed at an appropriate distance from each other, and that there is enough room for an adult male to place his foot between the rungs.

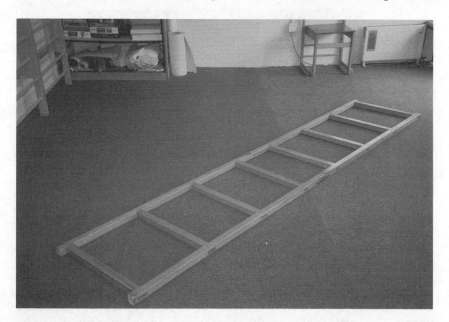

Fig. 6.6 Ladder

A ladder has particular significance for people with Parkinson's disease, as it provides a solid object for them to step over. This can, in some cases, enable the person to overcome freezing.

PARALLEL BARS

Figure 6.7 shows traditional parallel bars. These are a must for anyone working in a centre. The bars can be used in a variety of ways to teach balance, stepping and transference of weight. They enable the individual to maintain security while trying movements which may be difficult.

These bars should not be fixed but should be free to move if the person places too much weight on them. In this way the person can learn to find their balance point. If the bars are fixed then they will not be able to learn how to balance as there will be no feedback. The individual should not be placed in a situation where they will feel insecure, so the conductor must stay alongside them and assist them until they feel secure in a standing position.

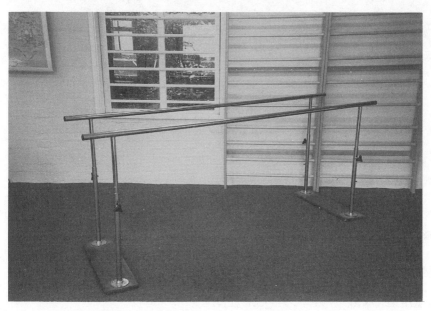

Fig. 6.7 Parallel bars

WALL BARS

Wall bars are useful if additional security is required. They are fixed and cannot assist in teaching balance, but can help a participant to experience an upright position.

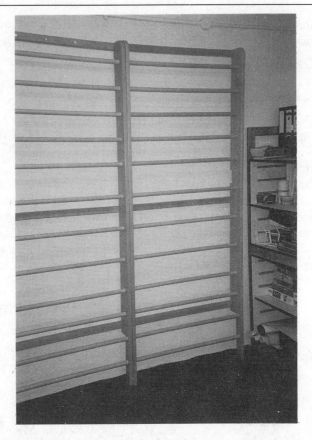

Fig. 6.8 Wall bars

The above represent the main pieces of traditional, wooden furniture which would be required in a centre teaching conductive education to adults. There are numerous items of equipment and aids available within the United Kingdom and the professional must be very clear about the use of this equipment before purchasing it.

ADDITIONAL AIDS AND EQUIPMENT

As a general rule, the more complicated the furniture or aid, the less likely it is that the person will be able to access it outside the centre. If a participant is only able to use an aid at the centre to achieve a movement, then they will not be able to apply their learning to their everyday situation. In this instance learning will be reduced, and the aim will become one of exercise. This may have a place with certain people but the professional must be very clear about this possibility when using the equipment.

In catalogues there are aids designed with a very specific purpose in mind, and we have to find out whether that purpose is suitable for our situation. There are certain factors to help us when making these choices. Equipment or aids should:

- assist movement and not replace it
- be of a height where the individual can feel secure but not transfer their weight on to it
- be removed or reduced as learning takes place
- not solve a problem but enable learning
- be carefully monitored at regular intervals during use.

Unfortunately we often see aids that have become a part of daily routine: a foot splint that has become a part of a person's dress; a stick or walking frame that has become a part of life; splints that are worn all day. In some cases it is necessary to replace certain movements or use an aid, but this decision must be carefully monitored.

If we are looking at individuals with head injury, stroke or cerebral palsy, then we are working towards improving movements. A person who has suffered a stroke may have a dropped foot in the initial stages and a splint may enable them to take steps and thus increase independence. However they should also be learning how to regain control over their foot and this will not happen if they put their splint on when they get up in the morning and take it off at night. In this situation movements will become restricted and need to be replaced.

Alongside the use of aids there should be times when the person is learning the skills required to replace the aid. This may not always be possible, but time and teaching should be provided towards this end, and the aid should not be seen as the only solution to the problem.

APPROPRIATE USE OF AIDS

Today we all use aids and equipment which make our life easier; luxury items such as microwaves, remote controls, cars and electric can openers have all become a part of our everyday life. The person with a neurological condition is no different, the difference is in the choice. An able-bodied person may regularly use a car but can walk if necessary or get on a bus; they may use a microwave but can cook, or use a remote control but can get up and switch channels. If we enforce dependency on aids then we remove this choice from the individual.

If the person has a progressive condition, we may need to assess the use of aids to maintain movements as much as possible. Aids and equipment have a significant role in assisting the individual who has a motor problem, but they must not be seen as the only method of overcoming problems – learning also plays an essential role.

Equipment must be appropriate for the individual. Standard equipment may not always enable the person to use it in the most appropriate way. This is particularly true of walking frames or sticks. All too often the stick or frame has been designed to allow the person to transfer their weight on to it. In doing so, the person moves their centre of gravity away from their body. Figure 6.9 shows the long-term effect of this. A stick or frame used in this way will replace movement and not assist it, since the person will lose the ability to find their natural centre of gravity. Constant use of this aid will cause the centre of gravity to move away from their body with the result that standing up straight will make them feel as if they are falling backwards. This shift in the centre of gravity will, in the long term, increase dependency on the aid.

If, however, the aid is at an appropriate height, then the person will be able to rest their hands on it and feel secure. In turn, their balance will improve as they learn how to find and maintain their own centre of gravity. This is very important when working with adults, as much of the standard equipment available is often not high enough for this purpose. Generally they were designed with a different purpose in mind and often special equipment has to be ordered for adults.

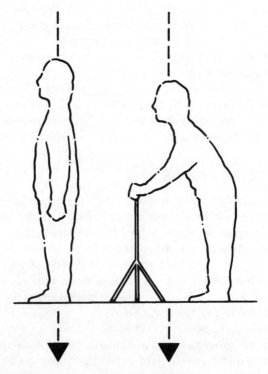

Fig. 6.9 Change in centre of gravity with use of aid

WHEELCHAIRS

Wheelchairs are now available in many different forms and can be individualized as necessary. Again, it is very important to be clear about the
aims when using them.

If the person is learning to control over-movements and is therefore
strapped into their chair for security when moving around, they will not,
during that time, be learning how to gain control of their limbs. If the aim
is to move from A to B safely, then these straps are playing an important
role. However, there should be times when the straps are removed, as,
without this, over-movements will increase when the body begins to use
the straps instead of the body as the limits of over-movement. All straps on
wheelchairs **must** be removed at certain times to allow the person to
increase their level of skill and should not be seen as controlling movements.

AIDS AND INDEPENDENCE

Equipment and aids should be as portable as possible. If equipment is only
available within the person's home then they will be de-skilled if they move
from this environment. The environment plays a large role in independence, and if the person is only independent in one environment, then
they are dependent on this environment. This will reduce social activities
and, in the long term, reduce self-confidence. If equipment is not portable,
an alternative should be found to assist the person outside their home and
the appropriate skills learnt alongside this.

When an individual attends for a consultation it is possible they will
have a number of aids which they use on a regular basis. The conductor
must discuss these with them and help them to find ways of using these
aids to assist movement and not replace it. In doing this, the conductor
must recognize that the person has probably become dependent on these
and will feel de-skilled if they are removed.

The relationship between a person and their wheelchair or any aids
which they use is very important. If they can be taught that aids enhance
skill, the participants often find that there is an increase not only in their
level of skill and independence but, more importantly, in their self-esteem
and self-confidence.

ORTHOFUNCTION

In conductive education we often hear the term **orthofunction**. This is a
new term for the western world, and one that has often been misinterpreted
to mean living without aids or adaptations. This is neither true nor practical. Many observers remark on the lack of aids in Hungary; this is not only
due to conductive education as a system but also to the lack of availability

of those aids and equipment we see in the United Kingdom.

Orthofunction means living with maximum independence and using full potential to achieve this. Aids and equipment do not enter into the concept of orthofunction, it is not a physical state but a stage in learning.

WHAT IS A TRUE AID?

The test of any aid is whether it can be removed. If it can, then it has served the function of assisting movement, but if it cannot then it replaces movement. Both of these roles are important, but the conductor should not encourage replacement of movement until all stages of learning have been explored.

To professionals and providers an aid has a very different meaning than for the user. The individual may feel that they have failed if they use an aid; many people attending the Institute have difficulty with walking, but will not use an aid because to them it represents failure. This should not be the case, but careful explanation is required so that the participant realizes that use of an aid can enhance performance and does not necessarily reduce it.

Reliance on an aid comes from lack of teaching; fear of failure comes from lack of teaching. The conductor must ensure that the individual does not have to face this; if it is felt that an aid is essential to replace movement, then this must be explained. An aid can assist with other skills and the emphasis should be placed on this.

Example

A young woman with MS came to the Institute for a consultation. She did not want to use an aid for walking because she was afraid that if she started using one then she would not be able to walk again, and that one aid would lead to another and she would end up in a wheelchair. At this time she was unable to move from room to room in her home. She could move around the room by holding on to furniture. Her movements were so restricted that she needed someone there to assist her to go to the toilet or to another room.

This fear was sensitively discussed with the conductor and her family and it was agreed that she would try to use a frame at home when moving from room to room. The frame would be left at the doorway of the room because she would be able to use the furniture. Alongside this, work was carried out within the sessions to improve her balance, posture and confidence. The frame was only required for a short time, she then began to use a stick and is now mobile around the house and able to walk more during the day. Within months she was able to walk without the use of an aid at home and with a stick outside. She now had independence and could safely be left alone in the house.

This is an example of how to use an aid to achieve the correct relationship between an aid and the user. Many children cry because the stabilizers on their bike have to be taken off and they no longer feel safe. This is a backwards step as far as they are concerned, but with encouragement and practice they are able to quickly ride their bike alone and are proud that they no longer use stabilizers. Aids should be used in a variety of ways to provide a means of achieving a goal and not to reduce goals.

PART TWO
Neurological Conditions

Parkinson's disease 7

This chapter outlines the main symptoms of Parkinson's disease and explores how conductive education is able to offer assistance to people with this particular neurological disorder. The chapter will include:

- a brief outline of the neurological damage caused by the disease
- the symptoms and manifestations of the disease
- an overview of drug treatment
- the consultation
- the planning of the conductive programme
- facilitation.

NEUROLOGICAL DAMAGE CAUSED BY PARKINSON'S DISEASE

In 1817 James Parkinson wrote an essay entitled, 'An Essay on the Shaking Palsy' (Parkinson's Disease Society, 1992). This paper is still recognized today as a classic description of the disease subsequently known as Parkinson's disease. In order to appreciate the nature of the disease, some knowledge is needed of how the brain works.

THE WORKING OF THE BRAIN

The nervous system consists of a complex structure of nerve cells and connections which combine to control bodily functions so that the whole body can respond to external stimuli (Stern and Lees, 1982).

The cerebrum is the most sophisticated structure within the brain and it consists of two large hemispheres. These act as an exchange, similar to our telephone exchange. The cells are referred to as grey matter and the fibres relaying the information as white matter. Within the cerebrum is a tissue that allows skilled and refined motor patterns to be executed.

The cerebellum lies behind the cerebrum and is often known as the little brain. The spinal cord is connected to the cerebrum by the brain stem. The brain stem processes nerve messages and connects with both the cerebellum and the cerebrum; thus it is an important link. The spinal cord nerve cells receive messages from higher centres in the brain and also pass on messages from the periphery. This is involved in the control of posture, balance in space and prevents overshooting of voluntary movements.

There are two main types of peripheral nerves, motor and sensory, that work together.

Motor nerves

Transmit instructions to the muscles, thus will control the state and movement of these.

Sensory nerves

Carry information about touch, pain, heat and position in space.

Some movements do not link with higher centres; if you put your hand on the stove and it is hot, you will automatically withdraw your hand. This is a reflex action controlled at spinal cord level. More complex movements require the intervention of higher centres.

The basal ganglia

Consist of large masses of grey matter located in the hemispheres. There are three sections to these: corpus striatum, globus pallidus and substantia nigra. The basal ganglia is considered important as a processing centre for movement information from the cerebrum.

In 1817 when James Parkinson wrote about the disease, it was impossible to examine the effect on the brain of the symptoms he was describing. He speculated that the damage was at the top of the spinal cord and the lower portion of the brain stem. In 1893, a doctor called Tretiakoff (Stern and Lees, 1982) examined the substantia nigra in people with Parkinson's disease and found that this was damaged. It is now generally accepted that other parts of the basal ganglia are also affected by the disease.

If we look at the way a nerve cell works, we see that it is a structure that allows the transmission of messages around the brain and the body. These do not directly touch each other but have a small gap called a synapse. The synapse is stimulated by the release of a chemical, called a neurotransmitter. These neurotransmitters have been recognized and many different ones can be found within the whole structure.

In the 1950s, a chemical substance called dopamine was found to be present in the brain. High concentrations of this were found in the basal ganglia. A pathway was discovered between dopamine-containing cells in the substantia nigra and cells in the corpus striatum. Parkinson's affected brains are known to contain very little dopamine in the basal ganglia. Dopamine was also found to regulate release of hormones influencing mood, behaviour and control of movement.

This is a very simple overview of the working of our brain and the role that dopamine plays. It should be not be seen as a comprehensive explanation of the neurological effect of Parkinson's disease, but as a guide to a greater understanding for those with little or no knowledge of neurology. We know that Parkinson's disease is characterized by a lack of dopamine, but the cause of this is still unknown. Much research has been undertaken in this field, but there has been no single cause found to date. Much of the research has concentrated on finding a cure for the disease and drugs to control symptoms, and great strides have been made in this area, for example Rinne Klinger and Staurm (1980) and Olanow and Lieberman (1992).

SYMPTOMS AND MANIFESTATIONS OF PARKINSON'S DISEASE

THE THREE DISTINCTIVE SYMPTOMS

The three distinctive symptoms of Parkinson's disease, as described by Caird (1991), are:

- involuntary shaking of limbs (tremor)
- stiffness of the muscles (rigidity)
- slowness and poverty of movement (bradykinesia).

These symptoms will naturally have very individual manifestations and degrees of disability. We know that Parkinson's disease is degenerative but there is no set pattern to this. It is generally thought of as an old person's disease, but this is not so. The onset of Parkinson's disease can be from the late teens, however the incidence increases during later life. About one in every thousand people in the United Kingdom will develop Parkinson's disease (Stern and Lees, 1982), and 75% of these will be between the ages of 50 and 75. Between the ages of 60 and 70, approximately one in every hundred people will develop this disease.

The incidence for men is slightly higher than for women and the disease seems to occur in a similar way throughout the world. There are few geographical differences, although it is less common in the black population of the United States, and in Japan there have been isolated cases of children developing it. In general, race or creed have no significant bearing on the incidence of the disease.

OTHER SYMPTOMS

In addition to the three symptoms mentioned above, there are a number of others. These are not necessarily secondary symptoms, and can appear in a mild or severe form. These symptoms and the manifestations and effects they have on the person and their personality are described briefly below.

Tremor

The tremor associated with PD is often called 'benign essential tremor' (Godwin-Austen, 1984). It usually affects one side and is most obvious in the arm or hand. It can, however, be seen in other parts of the body, particularly the head.

Tremor is present when the person is at rest, and often disappears when the limb is moved or used for active movement. Because of this, movements may not be hindered too greatly. This is a view held by, for example, Godwin-Austen (1984). McGoon (1990), a sufferer of PD, also comments on the personal effects of tremor. Tremor is rhythmical and generally quite slow, four to six times per second, but this is not standard and it may increase in speed.

One of the most significant effects of this symptom appears to be the social embarrassment caused by it. This is noted particularly with regard to stressful situations when there can be a significant increase in the tremor. We must not underestimate the social and physical effect that tremor of a limb can have upon everyday life.

Rigidity

The stiffness in muscles that is very common in PD can not only be disabling but also painful. It is often thought that there is no pain with PD, but this is not so.

Rigidity is a very severe form of stiffness: the muscles may actually feel rock hard and no amount of massage can release them. When moved passively, there is a resistance called the cog-wheel, which means that the muscles do not relax smoothly but as if they are moving along a circle of ratchets. This is more common when levels of dopamine are low, and in some cases drug treatment can help to overcome it. There are, however, always exceptions to this and it may be a condition which the person has to try and live with permanently. Rigidity of muscles severely affects the ability to take part in active movement.

Bradykinesia leading to freezing

Bradykinesia/hypokinesia is the medical term for a slowness of movements that can affect all actions including speech and facial expression. Slowness of movement does not just mean that the person needs more time; it is not a speed factor. The movement will become increasingly difficult to perform and more effort is needed to produce a diminishing movement. Movement may slow so much that it actually halts (freezing). This may happen at a most inopportune moment, for example when crossing the road.

The movement slows in a two-dimensional way, rhythm and amplitude, thus movements also become smaller. This is particularly noticeable with walking, when we see increasingly smaller steps and feet beginning to drag on the floor. Although the above example is very visible, all movements can be affected by this symptom – speech, breathing, facial expression, writing and everyday activities.

It is a very disabling symptom and one that is difficult to understand. We can all wait for someone who is slow, but the decrease in the amplitude of movement is frustrating for the person with PD as well as the onlooker. Again there may be no pattern for this, it may suddenly occur, and we have a scenario where one minute someone can perform an activity or movement and the next they cannot. This can be misunderstood as a lack of co-operation on the part of the person. The slowing down of movements may occur over a period of time but it can also happen very suddenly, with no warning.

Postural changes

The typical person with PD posture includes bent knees, hunched shoulders, elbows bent and lack of spontaneous arm movements. This posture can be seen in Figure 7.1.

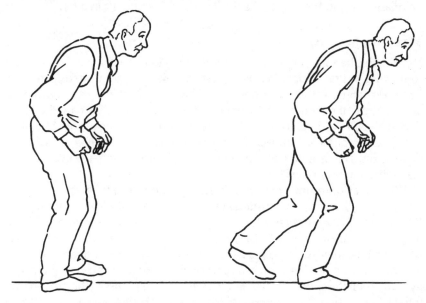

Fig. 7.1 Hurrying gait of advanced Parkinson's disease. (From a drawing by Paul Richter, in Stern, G. and Lees, A., *Parkinson's Disease. The facts*, 1982, by permission of Oxford University Press.)

This so-called 'typical' posture is not often seen, and usually only when dopamine levels are very low.

There are, however, many other postural problems associated with PD. If a person has a tremor on one side of their body, they automatically remove the weight from this side, thus leading to a tendency to lean to one side. This will have a direct affect on the ability to balance in both sitting and standing position.

If dyskinesia is present, the person will adopt a posture to enable them to retain control over their limbs, and this is likely to cause them to move their limbs behind their centre of gravity. Weight is often borne over the heels, again making balance difficult. As the position of the limbs changes, so does the position of the head in order to maintain an equilibrium, so the head is often tilted to one side.

The person with Parkinson's disease may be totally unaware of these postural changes and will need external advice about the corrections to be made. Problems with posture have the greatest knock-on effects on balance and movement.

Retropulsion

This can occur in any direction and is particularly noticeable when walking downhill. The movements increase gradually in speed and the person may be unable to stop them voluntarily. This can often result in a fall.

Mask-like facial features

Despite this being a very common symptom, James Parkinson did not refer to it in his initial paper (Pentland, 1987). This symptom often leads to a misinterpretation of the personality of the individual and can compound an impairment of speech, thus leaving the person socially isolated.

Facial expression is fixed, so that the person may appear bored, hostile, sad, angry or passive. Humour may appear as sarcasm due to a lack of facial expression. The face may also have a 'greasy' complexion, the eyes tend to stare and blinking may be reduced.

When we communicate with others, we tend to use their facial expression as an indication of their interest and opinion about what we are saying. If when talking to a person living with Parkinson's disease we receive a 'blank' expression, then it is easy to assume either that they don't understand or that they no longer wish to continue with the conversation. We also mimic each other's expression: if someone laughs, smiles or their eyes light up, then the speaker will respond with enthusiasm. On the other hand, if the listener shows no expression, then the speaker, in their turn, will also adopt this expressionless facial feature. The person with PD will see this and feel that the person no longer wants to speak to them, and this leads to a reduction in self-confidence. They may not be aware that they are seeing a mirror image of their own expression, as they are unaware of their expression. The internal expression is intact, they will feel as if they are responding appropriately since the problem is not an emotional one but the physical act of producing the movement they want to.

This symptom is perhaps one of the most disabling to the whole personality of the person, and one of the most difficult for the family to understand. It is almost without exception that we hear personal accounts of lack of interest, lack of motivation, loss of confidence, cutting off from social situations and depression, suggesting that much of this stems from the lack of facial expression and the image portrayed by the person as a result of this.

Reduction in gesture

Again, this is a very common symptom that may not appear to be very disabling but leads to a misinterpretation of social situations. In addition it can exacerbate the problem of stiffness. Lack of any spontaneous movement means that the person holds one position for considerable lengths of time, leading to stiffness – the same as we often feel when we get out of the car following a long journey.

Difficulties in writing

This has been mentioned above in relation to bradykinesia. Letters become increasingly smaller, and often the lines begin to slope downwards and tail off. This is known as micrographia (Figure 7.2).

There is also another form of writing difficulty not directly associated with PD – one that appears as a result of the side-effects of the drugs taken. This writing formation shows signs of dyskinesia. The letters are very difficult to form and take on an unusual shape, making it very difficult to read. This style has the appearance of 'untidy' writing and may be illegible (Figure 7.3).

An inability to write legibly means that a form of communication cannot be accessed, and whilst we have many machines to help with this, they are not suitable in all circumstances. If the signature is affected, as it often is, then it can be very awkward for the person if they are paying by cheque or credit card. Loose change is difficult to pick up. As a result the person often finds that they have to ask someone else to take control of their financial independence.

Speech/Breathing problems

Speech tends to be monotonous and lacks volume and intonation (Scott, Caird and Williams, 1985). This makes it uninteresting for the listener and, coupled with lack of facial expression and gesture, the person often feels a

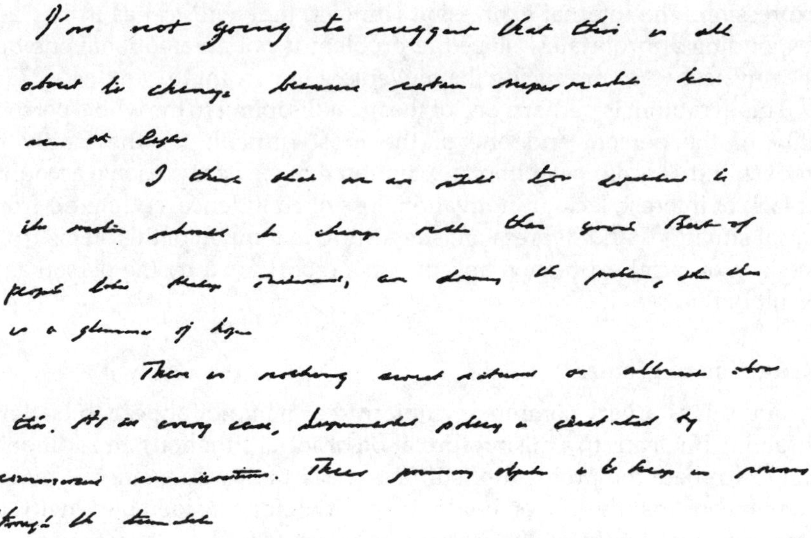

Fig. 7.2 Example of micrographic writing style

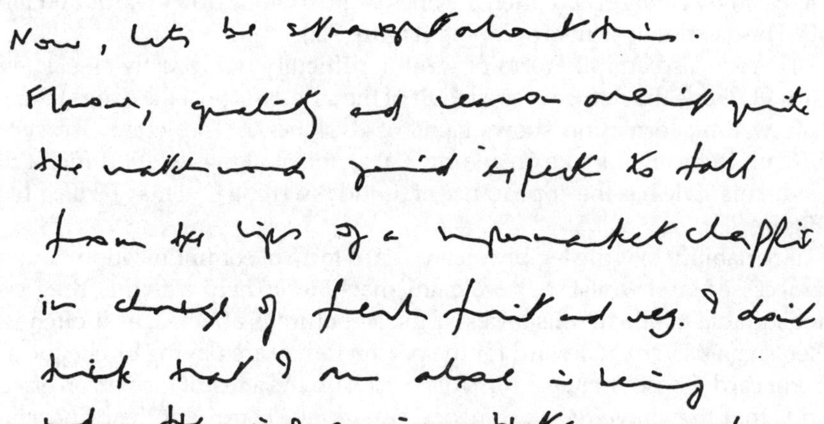

Fig. 7.3 Example of dyskinetic writing style

social outcast. In addition to this, the problems with initiating movements mean that it is very difficult to take part in a conversation. By the time the person has been able to initiate his speech, the conversation has moved on or their statement is no longer appropriate.

Breathing may become very shallow and so breath may run out before the person has finished speaking. This means that sentences are no longer fluent and it can be difficult to establish the meaning of their conversation. Pauses for breath may be in an inappropriate place thus breaking up the sense of what is being said.

Dribbling

This naturally causes great problems socially. It can also be coupled with difficulty in swallowing. The lack of voluntary swallowing that controls saliva flow is reduced, therefore saliva collects and begins to dribble.

Loss of concentration

It is difficult to ascertain whether this is a side-effect of the drugs or a symptom of the disease. Again, this causes many problems and is distressing for the person concerned and their family.

Problems with continence

These problems are not necessarily due to loss of bladder control but to the fact that the person may not be able to get to the toilet in time due to a slowness of movements. In addition, it is quite common that following a period of a lack of dopamine and immobility, the bladder begins to work before the person is able to produce voluntary movements, thus the person needs to empty their bladder but is unable to walk to the toilet to do so.

Rigidity of muscles can also occur in the bladder, and the person may find that they are unable to relax the bladder enough to enable them to empty it even though they know that they need to. The same can be true of the bowels and can lead to constipation, often made worse by certain anti-parkinsonian drugs.

DRUG TREATMENT FOR PARKINSON'S DISEASE

Drug treatment for PD is not a simple process; there are many drugs available and they play many roles in the treatment. Most people find that they take a cocktail of drugs which change as the disease progresses. Drug treatment controls the symptoms but does not treat the disease. As yet there is no known cure, so, depending on the symptoms and the level of the disease, drugs will be given accordingly.

There are no set patterns for the taking of drugs; these are often designed by the individual themselves in consultation with specialists. Once a daily regime is found that suits the individual they tend to stick to it until they feel that the symptoms are increasing or the effectiveness of the drugs is reducing.

Levadopa (Sinemet and Madopar)

These drugs directly replace dopamine that is not produced due to the disease. In the long term these drugs can lose their effectiveness and an 'on–off effect' occurs. This means that the person is able to benefit from the drugs for a period and then experiences a period where they are unable to move. This fluctuation can be directly linked to the timing of the drugs, however it can also be sudden and unexpected. This is very traumatic for the person because they are unable to plan their activities since they do not know whether they will be able to move or not. In addition, the person tends to try to do everything whilst they are 'on' and fatigue can result.

Selegiline (Deprenyl and Eldepryl)

These drugs prevent the breakdown of dopamine in the brain. They are often used alongside Sinemet and Madopar to enhance the effect, and can result in an increase in the time they work or a reduction in the dosage required.

Dopa-agonists (Bromocriptine, Lysuride, Pergolide)

These drugs stimulate the parts of the brain where dopamine works. They may be taken as a replacement for levadopa or in conjunction to try and smooth out the fluctuations.

Anticholinergic drugs (Artane, Disipal, Kemadrin)

These block the action of acetylcholine that causes a reaction with the lack of dopamine. They are generally not given to people over the age of 75 and are used less frequently now.

Apomorphine

This is usually taken in injection form or controlled with a pump. It helps to reduce the fluctuations in the levadopa treatment. It is used alongside other drugs and acts very much as a 'boost' as it is usually taken when the person is experiencing a severe 'off' period. It acts directly on the site of the brain where dopamine is active. The results of this can be quite dramatic but do not last very long.

This is not an exhaustive list of the drugs available but outlines the uses of the main types.

All these drugs have some side-effects whether this be dryness of mouth or constipation through to hallucinations and severe involuntary movements (dyskinesia). The balance of drugs against the level of side-effects is a very fine one and one which each individual has to find for themselves. For some the 'price' of dyskinesia is acceptable for them to be able to move around. For others the dyskinesia may be more distressing and painful than the Parkinson's disease symptoms themselves. It is mainly for this reason that each individual must find the drugs and levels that suit them and their lifestyles and personalities.

The side-effects of the drugs can increase the symptoms which one sees in PD, and it is sometimes difficult to know where the cause lies. In some cases the therapist has to work with two different diseases – one of a lack of movement, one of an increase in movement. This swing can happen within minutes. The drugs do not work along a nice smooth curve in all cases, but without them the person would quite quickly become very severely disabled.

THE CONSULTATION

Before attempting to work with someone with PD, the conductor must have a working knowledge of the disease and how it affects people. This will give the general picture that acts as a baseline. From this all individual manifestations are observed, including the side-effects of the drugs used.

APPLICATION FORM INFORMATION

Before the person attends for a consultation an application form will have been filled out, which will include the information described in Chapter 1 together with more diagnosis-specific information such as:

- present level and doses of drugs
- presence of tremor – when it started, in which part of the body
- presence of rigidity – when it started, in which part of body
- slowness of movements – established by asking about everyday movements, e.g. turning over in bed, standing up from a chair, dressing, etc.
- speech – problems to be specified
- side-effects from drugs
- continence of bladder and bowel.

The present level of drugs, including a history since diagnosis, is very important as it will give a general pattern of how the disease has progressed over time. The time between diagnosis and assessment is significant as a figure but by no means reflects the outcome of intervention. The conductor must assess the level of ability of the person and then look at areas where help can be given. The person also has the opportunity to express areas in which they would like help and these will be put together to form the basis of recommendations and possible provision.

INFORMATION AT CONSULTATION

From first introduction the conductor will be observing the spontaneous movement of the person – including posture, balance and size and length of stride. During this observation the conductor finds out whether there is a one-sidedness and the degree of this, and looks at use of gesture, speech ability and facial expression. This can all take place while the person is coming into the room.

The person then sits down and further information is gathered. This may be about the progression of the disease, the present difficulties, areas of concern, associated medical disorders, particularly if there are any heart problems. The conductor will have most of this information from the application form, however, there may be areas which need clarification.

Whilst discussion is taking place, the conductor can observe in more detail any speech problems, sitting posture and use of gesture. Tremor may be worse than usual due to the nature of the situation, and this needs to be taken into consideration. Any dyskinetic movements need to be observed and the intensity and areas of these noted. In addition the conductor will begin to notice techniques used by the person for controlling movements such as tremor or dyskinesia.

The participant is then asked to write down their name, address and a short sentence, and to sign and date the piece of paper. The paper used for this should be plain as this will give a greater indication of any writing difficulties. Any confusion or intellectual problems will also be highlighted here. This paper needs to be filed alongside the consultation notes for future reference.

Initial observation of movement

The conductor now needs to pinpoint any deformities or loss of range of movement. The participant will perform a few tasks in a lying position including movements that establish the range of shoulder, knee, elbow and hip movements. Basic movements, such as rolling to one side, sitting up and lying down are also carried out. These will show any signs of brady-kinesia, the ability to maintain and/or find a straight position, as well as general mobility. Tremor and/or dyskinesia will be observed, which areas of the body are affected, and to what extent.

At all stages the conductor must reassure the person, and if it appears that they are unable to perform the movement should help them to do so.

The conductor establishes when to help and when to stand back. This can usually be gauged from the person's reaction, in particular the look in their eyes. Lack of facial expression must be accounted for and not confused with a lack of understanding or disinterest.

Finer movements, hand–eye co-ordination and lower limb movement

The conductor will want to see finer movements and hand–eye co-ordination. The participant sits facing the conductor so that they can copy movements. They are asked to turn one palm over and then swap to the other. The conductor will change the rhythm of this, to assess the person's ability to maintain and change the rhythm of their movements. Movements such as bending fingers one at a time, lifting fingers and flicking fingers are also important to establish the range of movements of the person.

They will be asked to stand up from the chair and sit down again. From this the conductor can assess the point of their balance and whether this is behind, in front of or in line with the line of gravity. Throughout this, movements of other parts of the body, particularly the lower limbs and movements of alternate hands, as well as both together, are observed.

The conductor also assesses the ability to move lower limbs, and again this will be done in a sitting position. The person will be asked to lift their knees up, stretch their legs out in front of them, move the legs out to the sides and in front of them. Again, movements with a changing rhythm will be performed to discover any problems of initiating movements.

The conductor has been able to assess the range and rhythm of movements, the extent of bradykinesia, rigidity, tremor, speech and breathing, dribbling, writing, dyskinesia, use of gestures, intellectual ability and concentration. These are the main symptoms. The conductor may also ask specifically about continence and depression, if these are relevant, and enquire about the general daily routine of the person, including hobbies and interests. This all helps to build a picture of the personality of the individual.

Following all this, the conductor now needs to determine how conductive education can help the participant. Short-term goals are set in line with all the information received. The person is allowed time to consider these and to ask any questions. The carer/spouse can ask about anything relevant to their situation. A written report is sent to the participant within a few days.

This is the general outline for an initial consultation. The conductor must observe spontaneous as well as directed movements, try to get to know the individual and ascertain their needs within this time. This should take about an hour in total.

Having performed the consultation, the conductor must be aware that they have only seen one side of the person, as it is likely that they have used their drugs so that they are able to perform movements. There will come a time when performing them will be more difficult, and the conductor should show the individual that they are aware of this so that the person does not feel that they will always have to 'perform'.

Once they have begun attending sessions, the conductor needs to create the situation where they can observe all aspects of the participant's condition, including when drug levels are low. Any help given must include both the 'on' and the 'off' periods if it is to be of any use to the person throughout the day. The conductor should know for what percentage of the day the person is able to move, and for what percentage they experience bradykinesia or freezing.

PLANNING THE CONDUCTIVE PROGRAMME

There are two levels of programme planning – **general** and **individual**. The majority of work with people with PD is carried out in groups, since this helps to provide the stimulus needed to overcome problems of initiating movement. Thus a programme must be designed that allows each individual to benefit **within** the group.

A basic structure of tasks as described in Chapter 12 would be the starting place for each group. From here the conductor may wish to add or delete certain tasks. This cannot be done randomly as tasks must build on each other, and there must be a logic to the programme as a whole. In addition, there have to be short-and long-term aims, both covered by the task series. The programme is not a fixed structure, it will change according to the individual membership of the group and over time as changes occur.

OVERALL AIM OF THE PROGRAMME

It is important that the conductor is clear about the overall aim of conductive education for a person with Parkinson's disease. There is no known cure for the disease and it is of a progressive nature. Conductive education, therefore, cannot offer a cure; it aims to help the person to maximize the use of the movements they have, provides techniques to help overcome some of the symptoms, and encourages a positive, successful environment for the person, a learning environment. One observer to the Parkinson's disease groups at the Petö Institute remarked:

> The group reminded me of a class at adult education rather than at a physiotherapy/speech therapy session – a distinction which I think is important to make.

> (Baker, 1985)

One of the greatest factors with any progressive disease is the emotional level of the person concerned. This is remarked upon by many sufferers as being vital for physical well-being and the effectiveness of the drugs taken (Dorros, 1981). A negative emotional state leads to inactivity, this leads to loss of self-esteem and confidence, which in turn leads to further inactivity and depression. The conductor must help the person to achieve realistic goals; this will encourage them to try more and increase their confidence and self-esteem. This will lead to a positive attitude and an ability to play an active role in their own environment.

Parkinson's disease does not suddenly hit a person. They are almost waiting for the next symptom, the reduction in their abilities, and it is very important that they are helped to cope with this and, as much as possible, prepared in advance. Conductive education has a two-fold function for those with Parkinson's disease:

- to help overcome present difficulties
- to prepare the person with techniques they can use if and when required, i.e. a preventative role.

The conductor should have ideas for any problem the person faces and teach them techniques for overcoming them. The programme includes all the movements required for daily activities. There are a limited number of movements people make and these must be covered. As a general guide, we can start with the top of our head and work down to see what individual movements we are capable of – these should be included in the programme, the standard base for all programmes.

ELEMENTS PARTICULAR TO PARKINSON'S DISEASE

In addition the programme needs to include elements which are particular to Parkinson's disease. Complex movements of more than one limb are often difficult for people with Parkinson's disease, so tasks such as right hand on left shoulder and right heel on left knee may be included. Tasks that include changes in rhythm can also be difficult, so we may see making a fist with the right hand and changing to the left; the conductor sets the rhythm and changes this by increasing and decreasing it.

Specific tasks for writing are very important. These may take many forms and also serve a number of functions, such as helping to control dyskinesia or tremor, helping overall posture as well as directly helping the ability to write.

The tasks performed are not exercises. They are called tasks because they are not done to exercise muscles but to teach the appropriate movements. From this the person will put together these elements to help them perform the activity they wish, whether this be knitting, fly fishing or getting out of bed.

Functions are not taught as these restrict the individuality of the person. Each one of us performs a function in a different way that is very individual to us; the conductor, therefore, cannot impose their own individuality on the person.

Tasks are elements of actions used in everyday life, and the person with Parkinson's disease will, through the completion of the tasks, learn how to perform actions in the best way for them. This leads to control over symptoms but cannot remove or cure them.

There are specific elements that are helpful to the majority of people with Parkinson's disease, and these will be used throughout the task series.

- When sitting or lying, feet and knees are kept together. This helps to teach and maintain a central body position.
- Hands should always be fixed. This helps to teach control of tremor or dyskinesia. It also allows the person to adopt a symmetrical body position and thus helps with balance. The hands may be fixed on the hips, on the table, on the chair or wherever is comfortable for the person.
- Tasks are all performed with a strong rhythm. For any visitor to the session this is one of the most striking features (Cottam and Sutton, 1986). The tempo may change slightly according to the group.

  The person should be taught how to perform the movement on the count of one; this helps directly to overcome bradykinesia and the initiation of movements. This rhythm was discussed in more detail in Chapters 4 and 5.
- The conductor acts as a mirror image for the person, allowing them to have visual feedback of the movement they wish to do. This gives them a physical model of the movement to follow.
- All movements must be corrected by the conductor. In most cases this will be by verbal feedback, since the person will feel as if they are producing the required movement. This should be done in a positive but subtle way and should not lead to a feeling of failure.
- Movements should be carried out in as many positions as possible to maximize the opportunity for applying them.
- The participant learns to verbally intend and initiate the movement. Again, this allows them to use this technique and movement in other circumstances and not just during the session.

The conductor's main role is to lead the group, set out the tasks, and perform the tasks to allow the person to have an image of the required movement (naturally this is not possible for tasks in a lying position). In addition, as with all diagnosis, the conductor must facilitate both the individual and the group.

FACILITATION

There are many forms of this, each of which has been described in Chapter 1. The main forms used by the conductor for people with Parkinson's disease would be: educational, mechanical and rhythmical intention.

CHOOSING THE FORM OF FACILITATION

If we look back at the major symptoms of the disease, we will see that manual facilitation would not be of use to people with Parkinson's disease. If we consider rigidity and the cog-wheel symptom we can see that any manual help will increase the resistance of the muscle to activity and thus not produce the required result. Since many have a feedback loop which tells them that they are producing the movement, the conductor will tend to mainly use verbal facilitation; this may be in the form of correction, motivation, praise or encouragement. All of these are educational forms as they enable the person to learn how to achieve the desired movement.

It may be that manual facilitation is essential in order to maintain safety, and a conductor may hold a person's arm or hand whilst they are walking. The conductor will not manually perform the movement for the person as this will not enable them to learn the movement (Hári and Akos, 1988).

Many people with PD are able to perform a movement at certain times within their drug cycle, and they need to be advised of how to cope at the times when voluntary movements are more difficult. In order to achieve this, the conductor must first build up a mutual trust that enables them to help the person during their 'off' periods.

In addition to specific methods of facilitation the conductor needs to know when to stop or adapt a task series. This facilitates a positive environment and does not cause a loss of self-confidence. Each person must be helped to achieve a level suitable to them and their needs. They should never be asked to perform a task they are completely unable to do.

Thus the conductor facilitates the whole group by breaking down and building up the tasks, ensuring that tasks set for a whole group are relevant for each individual within it (Hári and Akos, 1988).

Example

The task is to put the hands behind the head. There will be some in the group who are able to do this, and there may be some who have severe rigidity and are unable to lift their arms further than their chest or forehead. These participants need to be made aware of what their task is before attempting it, and that in performing it they are achieving their aim. It is too late to explain this after the task since the participants will already have experienced failure.

Each individual will know their own potential and will therefore expect the conductor to also know this and to only ask them to perform within this. It would, however, be of no benefit to the group if everyone were to put their hands on their chest or head, as this would not allow everyone to reach their full potential. Thus the breaking down of tasks is very important.

Example

The conductor may want to build up a task for an individual or individuals within the group. Perhaps the task is to sit up from a lying position. For the majority of parkinsonians it is easier to sit up and swing straight to one side of the bed in one movement. if there are individuals who find this task relatively easy, then they may be asked to sit up forwards whilst maintaining straight legs, making the task more difficult for them. The main task will be the one that the majority of the group perform; from here the conductor will adapt when necessary.

It is important to remember that no facilitation is better than facilitation. Thus the conductor does not always need to correct the person; there will be movements they can achieve and these must be recognized more than movements that are more difficult to perform. This helps the conductor to maintain the balance between correction and the building of a positive self-esteem.

If a person with PD is having a really bad day (just the same as the rest of us may experience) when they are unable to switch 'on', then the conductor must allow for this during correction. It may be possible to correct everything but this will have no advantage for the person concerned. They, too, will know that their movements are restricted so any slight improvement must be encouraged. This is not patronizing, but recognition of the effort exerted and the outcome from this.

Thus the conductor is able to use facilitation to assist the person to achieve movements they would otherwise be unable to perform. The person must also be taught how to achieve these alone, and therefore facilitation should only be used if it can be reduced and eventually removed – with the exception of encouragement and praise!

SUMMARY

Parkinson's disease has many characteristic symptoms, the level and severity of which depend on the individual. The disease, although progressive, does not follow a set pattern.

The conductor needs to be aware of the person when they are 'on' and 'off', and the balance of problems in both states must be considered and built into the programme. The conductor must understand the disease and the side-effects of the anti-parkinsonian drugs. A positive, supportive learning environment should be built up for both the participant and their primary carer.

Conductive education cannot cure the disease nor prevent its progression. The conductor aims to help the person to overcome their difficulties, play an active role in their own rehabilitation and maintain the condition of the person for as long as possible by teaching them techniques they can apply in their everyday lives.

Drug treatment plays an important part in the lives of people with PD. Conductive education cannot replace drugs, but can help the person maintain this level at a minimum and, in some cases, allow them to reduce their dosages, thus decreasing the chance of side-effects. Individual patterns for taking drugs is discussed in the groups, allowing participants to learn from each other's experiences.

Multiple sclerosis

8

This chapter examines the main symptoms of multiple sclerosis and how conductive education is able to offer assistance to people with this neurological disorder.

The chapter includes:

- a brief outline of the damage caused by the disease
- the symptoms and manifestations of the disease
- an overview of the treatment
- the consultation
- the planning of the conductive programme
- facilitation.

DAMAGE CAUSED BY MULTIPLE SCLEROSIS

The pathological abnormality in multiple sclerosis (MS) is an area in which the myelin sheathing the nerve fibres has been damaged with relative preservation of the axons (De Souza, 1990). In later stages scarring occurs, and the lesion is then referred to as a plaque. These lesions are confined to the central nervous system and thus can be found in the brain stem, cerebellum, optic nerves and spinal cord; the peripheral nerves are not involved.

DEMYELINATION

The manifestation of the disease will depend on the site affected by demyelination – the name given to the process of destruction of the myelin sheath. The severity of the damage will vary between individuals and there are very few indicators to the prognosis for each person.

Possible areas of damage are:

Optic nerve	pain may be felt in the eye, eyesight may be blurred (return of central vision may take some weeks but is often complete in the initial stages).
Brain-stem lesions	may produce vertigo, loss of balance, in-coordination, diplopia, facial numbness, limb weakness, sensory impairment
Cervical spinal cord	loss of sensation in arm, ataxia, weakness and sensory loss in lower limbs, loss of sphincter control
Cerebral lesions	focal or generalized epilepsy, loss of intellectual functions, altered personality.

The cause of this demyelination is, as yet, unknown. There have been many suggestions, including hereditary, environmental and viral factors. There is, however, little consensus on these. In general, research has shown it to be primarily a disease of northern European races (Poser, 1984). The age of onset can range from less than 10 years to over 50 years, the average age of onset for both men and women being 29–33 years (Matthews, 1985). Statistics have shown that the relation of women to men affected is 3:2.

DIAGNOSIS OF MS

There is no single test that will confirm the diagnosis of MS; there has to be a combination of clinical history, symptoms and tests.

In 1983 (Forsythe, 1988) the Poser Committee laid down guidelines to assist with the diagnosis of 'definite' and 'probable' MS. This was done under two categories – clinical and laboratory-supported evidence.

Clinically definite MS

- Two attacks and clinical evidence of two separate lesions.
- Two attacks, clinical evidence of one and paraclinical evidence of another separate lesion.

Laboratory-supported definite MS

- Two attacks, either clinical or paraclinical evidence of one lesion and cerebro-spinal fluid (CSF) abnormalities.
- One attack, clinical evidence of two separate lesions and CSF abnormalities.
- One attack, clinical evidence of one and paraclinical evidence of another separate lesion, and CSF abnormalities.

Clinically probable MS

- Two attacks and clinical evidence of one lesion.
- One attack and clinical evidence of two separate lesions.
- One attack, clinical evidence of one lesion and paraclinical evidence of another, separate lesion.

Laboratory-supported probable MS

- Two attacks and CSF abnormalities.

An 'attack' is the occurrence of a symptom and/or symptoms of neurological dysfunction which last for more than 24 hours. These clinical features may remit completely or in part, may remain stationary for a prolonged period or may progress.

Poser (1984) identified 5 'types' of MS.

1. Relapsing and remitting – more than 70% of young patients begin with this form. The recovery after each attack is more or less complete. The frequency of these attacks is totally unpredictable.
2. Chronic progressive – 30% of all people with MS run this course from the onset. It tends to be more common in older people. Generally they exhibit the spinal form of MS and thus it is difficult to make a diagnosis.
3. Combined relapsing and remitting with chronic progressive – most people eventually have this form. They may begin with relapses and remissions but a chronic progression follows.
4. Benign MS – approximately 20% of the MS population exhibit this form. It means that there are very few inhibiting physical symptoms and a normal life span is expected. It is impossible to predict this form during diagnosis.
5. Malignant MS – less than 5 to 10% have this form, and it usually occurs in younger people. There are many severe relapses in the first year followed by a chronic progressive deterioration. These people can be severely disabled or even die within a few years of onset. Again it cannot be identified at diagnosis.

Laboratory tests

As mentioned, there is no one test that will confirm diagnosis, however there are certain tests that give indicators to the doctor to assist with diagnosis.

One of the main ones is examination of cerebro-spinal fluid (CSF), done by performing a lumbar puncture and withdrawing some of the fluid from the spine. Tests are then carried out to look for the presence of immunoglobin (IgG), which confirms that the problem originates in the central nervous system. Magnetic resonance imaging (MRI) is another common test for MS. This test can confirm the presence of lesions, although lesions alone do not prove a diagnosis of MS. Blood tests will exclude other possible diseases. Electrodiagnosis, as with MRI, can detect lesions; with the knowledge that MS tends to attack certain areas, then the following tests may be used: Visual (VEP) for the optic nerve, Brain-Stem Auditory (BAEP) for the brain stem and Somato-Sensory (SSEP) for the spinal cord–brain connections.

MS is therefore a difficult disease to diagnose, and following diagnosis there is little information that can be given to the person about the prognosis. There is no known cause to explain the disease and there is no known cure. The treatment and management of the person diagnosed with MS is a difficult, rocky ride for everyone concerned, particularly for the person receiving this diagnosis.

SYMPTOMS AND MANIFESTATIONS OF THE DISEASE

The multiple and varied nature of the progression of the disease make it very difficult to establish a set of symptoms. There are numerous individual variations leading to a complex set of symptoms.

PRINCIPAL CATEGORIES OF SYMPTOMS

There are however, nine categories of symptoms regarded as characteristic (Poser 1984).

1. **Visual loss in one eye**
    In many cases this is initially of a temporary nature. It can lead to a disturbance in orientation for the person as they are only able to see a part of the whole. It is also very frightening since the person does not know if and when the sight will return.
2. **Double vision**
    This could also be due to other causes. This symptom tends to come and go; there may be certain evident triggers, e.g. stress, hot weather, but it may come for no apparent reason. Again, it is usually temporary but can in fact remain permanent in some cases.
3. **Disturbance of balance and gait**
    This can take many forms. Balance may be affected by a weakness on one side, thus the person loses confidence and tries to compensate for this by using the other side. This inequality of weight distribution makes balance insecure. It could also be caused by ataxic symptoms where the body is unable to find and maintain a balanced position. Here the stance tends to be wide-based and steps are taken with straight legs. Both of these lead to an increased difficulty in walking where the person may 'drag' a weak leg behind them, may trip or may only be able to take a few steps before losing balance.
    In many cases aids to help with walking are given. These can alleviate problems of balance but may cause problems with gait. If a person is walking with two sticks then their weight will be distributed through their hands, which is why they have the sticks. Over a period of time they adopt a posture where hips are flexed, shoulders are in front of the centre of gravity, knees remain straight and are dragged through due

to the inability to lift them high enough. As balance becomes more difficult they will tend to splay their sticks thus giving them a wider base to increase security. Again, posture will be affected as they have to lean further forward.

Although walking aids are, in some cases, vitally important, the use of them must be carefully monitored to ensure that they do not add to the problems of balance and gait but help the person to maintain the posture they already have.

4. **Sensory disturbance in limbs**

This can mean that the person has little proprioceptive feedback from limbs. They may also be unaware of pain, changes in temperature, whether their shoes are on correctly, etc. It is very important that any limb that lacks sensory feedback, whether partial or total, is well monitored, and that the person is taught how to compensate for this loss. Without the correct advice they are subject to burns, pressure sores, skin and circulatory problems.

5. **Sensory disturbance in the face**

As with the limbs, it is important that the person learns how to compensate for the disturbance. This can also make eating and drinking difficult as well as giving the person a feeling of not 'looking' the way they expect.

If we think of the effect after an injection at the dentist and we are unsure if we are dribbling, we feel as if one side of our face is enormous. We think everyone sees what we are feeling, even though we can look in the mirror and know that it isn't so.

6. **Acute myelitis syndrome**

Inflammation of the spinal cord.

7. **Lhermitte's syndrome**

Tingling down the back and into the legs like an electric shock, produced by flexion of the neck. This is important for the therapist and family to be aware of. It is a very unpleasant feeling and this kind of movement should be avoided if possible.

8. **Pain**

This can be constant and makes each action or movement an effort. Pain killers may not relieve it. If someone is in constant pain, they will become withdrawn, move less and less, and are quite likely to be very irritable. Certain movements may incur more pain than others, and these should be avoided if at all possible.

9. **Progressive weakness**

This leads to uncertainty about abilities. The person is likely to wait when they wake up to see if they have the same strength as the day before. This weakness does not necessarily just gradually increase over a period of time, but can increase over a period of hours. Following rest, the original strength may have returned. Weakness tends to become apparent only when the person tries to do something that they used to be able to do and now no longer can. This is very distressing for both them and their families.

The person may experience one or more of these symptoms and the extent of this will depend on the number and position of the lesions. All the above are physical symptoms, but it must not be forgotten that there will be other complications associated with the diagnosis of a chronic progressive disease.

Poser (1984) identifies three areas of symptoms: primary, which in the main are included above; secondary, such as urinary tract infections, respiratory infections, pressure sores, contractures and nutritional problems; tertiary complications, such as financial, social and emotional problems, employment difficulties and, last but by no means least, the effect on family life and interpersonal relationships.

Broader categories of symptoms

McAlpine (1972) identified broader categories of initial symptoms and suggested the following incidence for the MS population:

- weakness in one or more limbs – 40%
- optic neuritis – 22%
- paraesthesia – 21%
- diplopia – 12%
- vertigo – 5%
- disturbance of micturition – 5%

Thus we can see that there is a fairly exhaustive list of possible symptoms for the person with MS. This list on its own will frighten people, even though they realize that they will not necessarily display all of these. There is, however, a lack of certainty, and this can cause some of the worst reactions to diagnosis. The fear of having all these symptoms is not only real but very understandable.

Psychological problems associated with MS

Simons and Aart (1984) explore the psychological problems associated with diagnosis of MS and see a conflict situation. On the one hand, the person tends to hide away from others and, on the other hand, there is a wish to be understood. This conflict is not only true of MS, it is one that is frequently reported by those diagnosed with any chronic condition.

Very careful handling is needed to assist the person to resolve this conflict. One of the most effective ways of doing this is to increase the information available to the general population, thus reducing the need for the person themselves to have to explain.

Fatigue

One symptom that has not been mentioned above, even though it is probably one of the most consistent, is that of fatigue. This fatigue is different from the tiredness that we may feel and causes many problems within the daily life of the person concerned.

When experiencing fatigue the person may be unable to physically move, they may not be sleepy but are physically exhausted. This often has to lead to a change in their daily routine and has a knock on effect on the family as a whole. It is not visible, not measurable and needs careful explanation to family and relatives as it can often cause many problems with home life. It can be misinterpreted as malingering, being unable to cope, giving up, etc. It is none of these; it is a very common symptom of the disease and one which can only be treated by developing a daily routine that allows for rest.

If the person with MS has a 'good' day and feels able to do all the things they want to, then it is possible that they will experience severe fatigue and have to rest for the next few days. This takes away the pleasure of having a good day and should be avoided as much as possible. There appear to be some triggers to this, such as warm climates or a hot bath, and this is why the person is often advised to avoid these.

We have seen that there are a wide variety of possible symptoms that may be experienced by the person with MS. There is uncertainty about the course these will take, uncertainty of the permanent nature of symptoms, uncertainty about the number of symptoms the person will actually experience and uncertainty about the disabling nature of symptoms. As many individuals as there are who are diagnosed, so there will be as many variations and degrees of severity of the symptoms.

TREATMENT AND MANAGEMENT OF MS

Treatment for MS is a very difficult topic. Since there is no known cause there can be no treatment for the disease itself, as this is reliant on the finding of a cause. In the meantime, treatment is based on the relief of symptoms aimed at reducing the suffering from the disease to enable the person to live more comfortably within their capabilities. This will include medical or surgical procedures together with varying therapies. This outline of the main areas of treatment and management should not be seen as an exhaustive list of possibilities.

When we are diagnosed with an illness or ailment we expect the doctors to provide the cure, the answer, the drugs to treat the problem. When the person with MS is diagnosed they are offered little hope in this area, and this invariably leads them to trying many different things in order to improve their condition. As a result of this, certain methods of treating symptoms have become widely accepted as useful by those with MS. These can be roughly placed in three categories: medical model, therapeutic model and alternative model.

MEDICAL MODEL

It is very common to hear of people with MS who receive steroid therapy. This can help to hasten the recovery from an attack. It is a little unclear how this works, but the input of these particular hormones often gives relief, sometimes quite dramatic, from the symptoms of an attack. This is particularly true at the beginning, although it appears that the effectiveness of repeated courses of this treatment decreases over time (De Souza, 1990), and in some cases the person may be totally unresponsive. From our experience with people with MS, it seems that there is some effect for three to four courses and after this very little or none. In rare cases a worsening of the condition has also been known.

Beta-interferon

One of the latest treatments, now undergoing trial in the United Kingdom, is beta interferon. The effects of this were in fact reported as early as 1981 (Jacobs *et al.* 1981).

Interferons are chemicals present in everyone, and they play an essential role in the immune system. There are three types of interferon – alpha, beta and gamma. Beta interferon inhibits the action of gamma interferon and it is thought that gamma interferon contributes to the destruction of myelin. Again, this offers no cure but gives hope to those who have the relapsing/remitting form of MS. The use of this drug is still in its infancy and as such only short term results are known.

Many people with MS have great hopes for this drug, quite naturally, but there are still medical reservations about its effectiveness. One of the big problems which has been reported in the press is the cost of this treatment. It is likely to cost around £10,000 per person per year, and there is a fear that there will be rationing due to the cost.

In 1995 a booklet was written by the MS charities in order to clarify the facts about this drug (Multiple Sclerosis Society, 1995). Here it was reported that people with the relapsing/remitting form should be considered for treatment and that trials were underway for those with the progressive form. If these were successful, then these people should also be recommended for treatment. This booklet also informs people that the NHS has not yet agreed to bear the cost of this treatment but that it can be obtained privately. This seems to be an ongoing argument for which no concrete solution has been found. Hopefully this matter will be resolved in the very near future.

In addition to the above drug-based treatments there is a surgical procedure that can help to reduce severe tremor. This involves surgically damaging a part of the contralateral thalamus to reduce the tremor; however this is very rarely performed due to the already progressive nature of the disease (De Souza, 1990).

Medical treatment can also be offered for secondary symptoms, such as urinary infections, swallowing problems, nutritional problems, and so on.

THERAPEUTIC MODEL

The medical model offers some degree of relief from symptoms; the therapeutic model, however, can have a wide range of functions. Its main role is to help the person to live the life they choose at each stage of the disease, i.e. within their capabilities. By definition, this means that the management of MS has to be both long term and flexible enough to account for the fluctuating nature of the disease.

Ashburn and De Souza (1988) suggest nine concepts for chronic care.

1. Long-term management.
2. Early referral.
3. Regular assessments to allow early identification of new symptoms or changes in existing symptoms.
4. Positive attitude by therapists to emphasize abilities and achievements rather than disabilities and handicaps.
5. Correct information accurately presented to help MS patient understand the disease and how their body reacts.
6. Patient responsibility fostering a self-help attitude to treatment.
7. Continuity of care for the individual patient ensured between all professionals involved.
8. Accurate and regular communication between team members, the person with MS, their families and carers.
9. Total overview of patient management achieved by professionals with sound knowledge of the condition and factors influencing it.

Therapy on a regular basis can assist in providing a feeling of well-being for the person with MS, and has a psychological benefit alongside any physical gain. This is very important for the person living with a progressive condition, and the therapist should ensure that maximum advantage is obtained in addition to any preventative measures that may be taken. Therapy should help the person to remain as active as possible for as long as possible.

ALTERNATIVE MODEL

Under this title we should include homeopathy, diet, hyperbaric oxygen and any other therapies or treatments that do not come under the 'conventional systems' used in this country. These are usually provided either by a charity or privately funded by the individual. It is impossible to look at all these in detail and explore the benefits of them for each individual; however they play a large part in the life of a person with MS.

In the absence of a cure or a medical or therapeutic model that has concrete and long-lasting effects, the individual will try as many things as possible until they find the ones which offer them some benefit. This benefit may not be measurable to the outsider but only to the person concerned.

Forsythe (1988) talks about the problem of scientific approaches as failing to see the importance of the uniqueness of the individual concerned. She also goes on to say that whatever the individual chooses to do it must be because they want to do it and that they feel that they benefit from it. It should not be seen as another chore but something that gives them some pleasure.

The range and benefits of the treatment and management of MS will vary according to the individual manifestations of symptoms and the range of services available. All professionals in this field, together with all those with MS, will be working towards increasing the quality of life for the individual for as long as possible, and at the same time working towards finding a cure for this disease. Much work is being done in these areas and the reader should familiarize themselves with both research and approaches to management in more detail.

THE CONSULTATION

As with any neurological problem, the conductor must first be aware of the possible manifestations of the disease for the individual attending for consultation. It is also important to know how the person rates their abilities on the day of the assessment. This is of particular importance when considering the fluctuations in abilities with MS.

The timing of the assessment is also important with regard to factors such as fatigue and weather. If it is a hot day then the person is unlikely to be able to perform many physical movements, the same is true if it is late in the day. These factors must be taken into consideration and the consultation performed accordingly. It is also possible that the person has had to travel a long distance to come to the centre. This can also have an effect on their abilities, as they may be fatigued or very stiff from the journey.

APPLICATION FORM INFORMATION

Before attending they will have completed an application form containing the general information described in Chapter 1. In addition to this, more specific questions will have been asked which are pertinent to the diagnosis:

- steroid treatment received
- presence of stiffness, in which limbs, when did it start
- presence of tremor, where, when did it start
- loss of sensation, partial or total, where, when did it start
- continence problems, frequency, bowel movements, ability to control continence, use of catheter
- main method of moving around: wheelchair, sticks, holding on to furniture, alone, etc; distinctions should be made between indoors, outdoors and long distances
- speech, problems to be specified
- writing, problems to be specified
- vision, problems at any time to be specified and dates given if possible
- all therapies, diet, etc; basic details to be given
- fatigue.
- an overview of general abilities with everyday tasks, washing, dressing, eating, drinking, etc.

This information will give the conductor an overview of the main problems and the rough progression of the disease. The time between diagnosis and consultation gives the conductor a base but will not reflect outcome, since there will be as many individual manifestations of the disease as there are people who come for consultation. Each person must be seen as an individual and the consultation should allow the conductor to establish short-term aims for that person.

INFORMATION AT CONSULTATION

From the first introduction, the conductor will be able to observe the spontaneous movement of the person. This is particularly important for those with MS as it is possible that due to fatigue they will not be able to perform many physical movements. In addition, it is possible that the person may be able to perform a movement in an isolated situation very well, but will be unable to use it in their everyday movements. The conductor is mainly concerned with the application of movements into everyday activities and not with movements in isolation, therefore it is very important to observe spontaneous movements.

Following introduction, the person is invited to sit down and the conductor will discuss with them in more detail any aspects arising from the application form. They will also be asked what they would like, what areas of concern they have and what help they would like.

It is important to ensure that the conductor balances information from both the individual and the prime carer or family member. The conductor needs to create an atmosphere where the person feels that they can discuss their problems, show that they understand these as much as is possible for an outsider, and that they want to help the person overcome their difficulties. This discussion should be realistic as it is just as damaging to give false hope than to give no hope at all. The conductor must remain factual but empathize with the person's situation.

As is true of all of us, they want to hear the truth and this can be presented in two ways – negatively or positively. The conductor must ensure that throughout the assessment they maintain a realistic but positive stance on the individual's problems and shares this information with them. The emotional effects of having a progressive disease for which there is no known cure or cause should not be underestimated. The individual needs to be treated as a person who has MS and not an MS person.

Assessing movement

Following this discussion, the conductor will ask the person to perform a few basic movements, that will allow the conductor to assess any deformities, contractures, the extent of spasticity and ataxic movements, their range of movements, and give them a guide to the abilities of the person.

The movements requested will depend on the overall level of severity of the condition. The person may be asked to lift their legs whilst sitting and lying, or perhaps just whilst lying. The conductor needs to ensure that the person is only asked to perform the tasks that they are able to try, and not those that are impossible for them.

The person may have great disorientation as a result of MS and may be afraid in a lying position. If this is so, then the conductor should immediately transfer the person to sitting. They may be able to sit on their own chair but feel very unsure on a chair without arms, again this has to be taken into consideration.

The person then returns to the table to discuss with the conductor how conductive education will be of benefit to them, what the short-term aims would be and specific areas of concern that may be helped.

During the consultation the conductor will have been able to look for the main symptoms associated with the condition, other specific information or problems may have emerged, and the conductor will have had the opportunity to learn a little about the personality of the person. This gives a good base for the conductor to move on to planning the programme or deciding which group would be the most appropriate for the individual.

This report and the results of any discussions will be followed up in writing to the person, since it is very common to be unable to remember the details of conversations.

This is the general format for a consultation with a person who has MS. There will be individual variations, but the conductor needs to find out the information presented above in order to decide how the person would benefit most from this form of provision.

PLANNING THE CONDUCTIVE PROGRAMME

As with all conditions, there are two levels of programme planning –
general and individual. Conductive education uses the group as a tool for
facilitating movement and success. However, in certain cases an individual
may prefer to be alone or may have a severe lack of movement and require
an intensive input.

THE BASIC PROGRAMME

Whether the person has an individual session or joins with others in a
group, the basic programme will be the same. Chapter 12 provides an
example of this programme that would be the base for the conductor, and
they may wish to then add or delete tasks. The programme is not fixed and
can vary according to the individual membership of the group. It may also
vary if some members of the group feel that they have come across a specific
problem since their last visit and would like some help with this. In
addition, factors such as heat may have an influence. Thus the programme
should not be seen as a rigid document but a strong base from which to
work.

   Conductive education cannot offer a cure for MS, but it can offer a base
for learning new movements or relearning ones that are now very difficult.
The aims of the programme are the same as those for other rehabilitation
methods. For example ARMS (Action Research for MS) suggest the following as guidelines for treatment:

1. Encourage development of strategies of movement.
2. Encourage learning of motor skills.
3. Improve the quality of patterns of movement.
4. Minimise abnormalities of muscle tone.
5. Emphasise the functional application of therapy.
6. Support the patient to maintain motivation and co-operation and to
    reinforce therapy.
7. Implement preventative therapy.
8. Educate patients re. the above, for coping with everyday life.

(Forsythe, 1988)

These guidelines would be very similar to those given to a conductor, the
ways of approaching them would, however, differ. The one exception may
be the use of the word 'patient', since this tends to imply that they will be
passive and will be treated. In conductive education they must play an
active role, be a partner, thus we tend to use the term 'participants'.

   The following is a quotation from a paper prepared by a visitor to the
Petö Institute in Hungary. It is an extract from a report submitted to the
British Council.

The teaching was very much geared to helping the individuals develop their own method of achieving function. The exercises were certainly not gymnastics but a means of re-achieving movement and, of course, there is a great mental component to the whole thing, with the body being subordinate to the mind.

(*Hayward, 1985*)

Thus the conductive programme aims to teach the person how to perform movements, how to overcome difficulties by teaching all the components of the movement skills needed. This then allows the person to call on these components when required. It is impossible to teach functions since the damage caused by the lesions will vary so much that abilities will not be uniform. Also each person will perform skills in an individual way which they developed before the onset of MS.

Conductive education has a two-fold function for those with MS:

- to help overcome present difficulties
- to prevent the onset of further problems as much as possible, and equip the person with techniques they can use if needed.

ELEMENTS PARTICULAR TO MULTIPLE SCLEROSIS

In addition to the basic programme, the programme for those with MS must include elements particular to MS and to the individuals within the group. The following is a list of ideas of possible elements needed in a task series for participants with MS.

- **Tasks to assist the reduction of spasticity**
  In general all tasks can do this provided they are completed in a slow rhythm. The person must have the time to initiate and perform the movement without causing spasticity to increase. This is a very difficult element for the participants to learn, but one that is vitally important. In addition there may be specific tasks, such as lying on the stomach and alternating movements, e.g. bending and stretching, that will help to reduce stiffness or spasticity.
- **Tasks to improve the aim of movements**
  This is particularly relevant to those who have signs of ataxia. All movements need to be started from and end in a fixed position. This way the person learns how to control their movement. Movements should be broken down into small stages to allow for a smooth transition from one stage to the next. Tasks such as putting finger to nose, on eyebrow, fist to forehead, etc. all help to teach an accuracy of movement together with increasing the awareness of the body in space.

- **Breathing tasks**
  This is very important as congestion of lungs and breathing difficulties are often associated with the later stages of the disease. If someone is a wheelchair user and unable to move spontaneously, then it is very important that they are taught how to increase and/or maintain their lung capacity. This will have an additional benefit for speech and circulation.

  Another important function of breathing tasks for a person with MS is that of improving continence. Frequency of going to the toilet is often a problem, one which can be helped by correct breathing. The participant is taught how to breathe into their chest and then push the air into their stomach whilst relaxing their bladder. This breathing technique has changed people's lives, offering them more freedom of movement and a more restful sleep. Breathing also has a known relaxing effect and can help to reduce spasticity and severe stiffness.

- **Visual tasks**
  There may be a problem with double vision or nystagmus. Tasks that teach how to fix the movement of the eyes, such as looking at the tip of a finger, focusing and then looking to a point further away and focusing, or following movements with the eyes only, etc. can have a positive effect on vision.

- **Tasks using other parts of the body**
  If the person has paralysis of the limbs as a result of the lesions caused by MS, then specific tasks would be required to teach them how to 'swing' in order to produce movement. This involves learning how to use other parts of the body to produce the required movement.

Example

If the legs are completely paralysed, then the person learns how to turn to the side and use the swing of the hips to produce movement in the lower limbs. This is particularly useful if the person wants to move in bed. It will not give them back their movements, but teaches them how to perform some voluntary movements that can help to reduce pressure sores or stiffness.

Whilst performing any of the tasks above, there will be some specific elements helpful to all participants. These will be used throughout the task series and become an integral part of the programme. These are the elements the conductor needs to observe; they are essential to the working of the programme and the tasks mentioned above.

The tasks themselves are not conductive education, they are one element of the whole. Another element is the methods of execution listed below.

- When sitting, lying or standing, feet and knees are parallel to hips.
- Weight should be evenly distributed on both sides of the body.

- Tasks should be completed in a symmetrical way.
- All appropriate tasks should be performed with right, left and both sides of the body.
- All movements should be performed by using the full range of movement for each individual.
- Movements should start from a correct basic position – this will vary in a lying, sitting and standing position.
- Movements should be executed in the given rhythm.

Basic positions

As mentioned above, all movements should start from a basic position. This position is to help with symmetry of movement and balance and control.

- Lying position – supine, legs stretched hip width apart, toes turned up, arms by side, palms facing down, head in midline.
- Sitting position – feet flat on floor, weight over whole of sole, feet and knees in line with hips, toes facing forward, shoulders back, head in midline, back straight, weight distributed equally over both hips.
- Standing position – hips, knees, feet in one line, shoulders back, arms relaxed by sides, toes facing forward, weight over both feet, knees stretched.

FACILITATION

One of the main methods of facilitation is rhythmical intention. In addition to this, the conductor needs to provide a very positive atmosphere for learning. Each individual must be given a technique to perform each task that allows them to experience success. This helps to create the positive atmosphere.

As well as educational facilitation, the conductor has to provide some manual facilitation. It must be stressed that this should not be the first type of facilitation used, but it will be necessary in some situations.

There is no manual facilitation designed especially for the person with MS. Facilitation is described in Chapter 1 and its principles are the same irrespective of the specific diagnosis. If the reader is unsure of how to help a person with MS achieve a task, they should refer back to this chapter.

SUMMARY

We have read that MS has a complex set of symptoms and a varying rate of progression. Conductive education, unfortunately, cannot reduce damage already present in the myelin sheath, but it can help the person to learn techniques to enable them maintain an active lifestyle.

The conductor needs to be aware of problems such as fatigue and sensory loss and assist the person in overcoming these. The task series can increase stamina and reduce levels of fatigue.

For any condition for which there is no cure, good management becomes the key issue in rehabilitation. The person with MS is able to learn motor skills that will assist in the overall management of the condition. A positive, supportive learning environment needs to be created to enable the participants to share experiences.

Traumatic head injury　　9

This chapter outlines the manifestations of traumatic head injury and the implications for those working with people with head injury within conductive education.

The chapter includes:

- a brief outline of traumatic head injury
- manifestations of neurological damage
- the consultation
- the planning of the conductive programme
- facilitation.

OUTLINE OF TRAUMATIC HEAD INJURY

Traumatic head injury is a term given to any form of direct injury to the brain. There are two main types.

Open head injury

Open head injury is perhaps the least common in the United Kingdom. This refers to injury such as gun shot where there is a point of entry and exit. This type of head injury will be more common during times of war than in peacetime.

Closed head injury

This type of injury occurs when the head has come into contact with an object. This is the type this chapter will be concerned with, and any further references to head injury will assume a closed head injury.

There are two forms of brain injury – primary, which occurs at the time of impact, and secondary, which occurs as a result of breathing difficulties, haemorrhage, etc. These need to be seen together to give a full picture of the damage caused by head injury.

CAUSES AND INCIDENCE OF HEAD INJURY

There are a number of causes of closed head injury. The following is not an exhaustive list but a list of the most common causes.

- road traffic accidents
- sports injuries
- alcohol related injuries
- fits and other causes of loss of consciousness
- assault
- falls
- domestic accidents
- industrial accidents.

Headway, the National Head Injuries Association, comments that every year one million people in Britain attend hospital with head injuries. This is a rate of 20 people per hour. Of these many are mild, and only 10% will have more severe problems that require intensive rehabilitation. The incidence in rates for males exceeds that in females in all age groups under 65 (Giles and Clark-Wilson, 1993).

SEVERITY OF HEAD INJURY

The severity of the injury is normally described in terms of the length of coma or post-traumatic amnesia. Wood and Eames (1989) identify seven groups of severity of head injury. The extent of the injury will have an effect on the outcome of rehabilitation, and therefore it is important for the conductor/therapist to be aware of the different levels of severity.

Group 1   The mildly or moderately injured who make rapid and complete physical recovery.

Group 2   Those with injuries of any degree of severity who have significant physical or communication disorders that are slow to resolve.

Group 3   Those with very long term coma and very severe physical deficits.

Group 4   Those with severe physical disorders who also have disorders of behaviour sufficient to make them unmanageable or unresponsive in standard rehabilitation settings.

Group 5   Those with injuries of any severity who make reasonably good and rapid recoveries physically, but who have severe changes in behaviour that make them unacceptable in standard social or treatment settings.

Group 6   Those who have suffered one or other of the very diffuse brain insults – hypoxia, ischaemia, hypoglycaemia or encephalitis with brain swelling.

Group 7   Victims of head injury whose brain injury is so severe that they never recover what may properly be called consciousness and remain in a persistent vegetative state (PVS).

Head injury of any form affects both the individual and the family. There are three main stages which the family have to go through, the first one being the life or death crisis. The person may be in a coma for hours, days or months. At this stage the important question is whether they will survive or not. Very little consideration is given to the outcome of the head injury. Following this comes the second stage where the person is beginning to reach consciousness – at this stage the effects of the head injury become apparent and it becomes obvious that there will be a long period of recovery. The third stage will be when the person goes home. Now the care that was given in the hospital falls on the shoulders of the family and the reality of the problems start to hit as the family are often caring for 24 hours a day.

REHABILITATION

Once medical care is no longer required full time, then the person is ready to move into rehabilitation. The forms and extent of this will vary according to the damage and the individual. Wood and Eames (1989) define the rehabilitative process in the following way:

> Rehabilitation is a process of teaching skills and abilities to individuals with physical and/or mental handicap. This implies a process of learning on the part of the patient, yet the apparatus which mediates learning, the brain, has been damaged and therefore the learning mechanisms cannot be assumed to be operating efficiently. The salient factors approach to brain injury rehabilitation is an attempt to collect information about the nature of an individual's brain injury in order to understand how the learning system of a brain is operating.

The label 'head injury' is therefore too vague as a basis for rehabilitation. If we consider that our brain is the control area of our very being, including physical, cognitive, communication and emotional areas, then injury to the brain can have any number of effects.

A starting point is to identify the main area of the brain affected as this will give some indication of the effects. As a general rule, people with injury to the frontal lobes may display personality changes bringing social handicaps that prevent them from exercising their physical abilities. Damage to the brain stem may result in severe physical deficits.

Whilst this gives us a broad outline of major areas of damage, we cannot assume that damage to the brain is concentrated in one area only. This is particularly true if we refer back to the main causes. Road traffic accidents for example are likely to produce multiple injuries, including those of the brain. Although it is usually the front (frontal lobes) or back (brain stem) of the skull which receives the impact, we must also allow for the possibility of damage to both, for example, the front of the skull may come into contact with a vehicle and the back may come into contact with the road.

Damage due to traumatic head injury is therefore very difficult to define, and time is usually required for the full extent of the damage to come to light. For this reason caution must be used when predicting outcomes and the benefits of rehabilitation.

Garner (1990) gives the following prognosis of the effects of rehabilitation following head injury. The age refers to the age at the time of the head injury.

Under five years may take decades
20–40 years   improve for up to five years
40–60 years   improve for up to two years
60+   cease to improve within nine months.

These are presented as a guide and the author offers no definition for the term 'improve'. Guides such as these can be misleading to the person concerned, the family and the therapist. Whilst it is accepted that greater recovery may happen during these periods, recovery will continue to a lesser degree throughout the person's life. The impact of smaller steps may be insignificant to the therapist but could mean far more to the person and their family.

We all learn something new every day of our life. The information learned may be important to us and trivial to someone else, but this does not mean that we cannot count it as a gain in knowledge. The head injured person is no different; they will continue to learn in some form throughout the period following their accident. What we have above is a guide for rehabilitation, and figures such as these should only be used within this context.

MANIFESTATIONS OF NEUROLOGICAL DAMAGE

In this section we are concerned with the symptoms following severe closed head injury. There will be an enormous variation in the degree and number of symptoms shown. Each person will be unique in the clinical picture they present and individual assessment is of vital importance.

Several groups of symptoms/damage may be present in one individual. The main areas where damage may occur are: motor deficits, communication problems, sensory problems, behavioural disturbances and cognitive problems. Broadly speaking, any aspect of human development can be affected to varying degrees by head injury. Thus by definition a wide variety of professionals will be involved with the head-injured person.

OVERVIEW OF SIGNS AND SYMPTOMS

The following is an overview of the possible symptoms and the manifestations of these. It is not an exhaustive list, but aims to summarize the main problems that the conductor/therapist must take into consideration when working with a person with severe head injury. Those with mild head injury should make a quick recovery and would not require long-term rehabilitation.

Aphasia Loss of ability to communicate. It may affect the ability of the person to speak (expressive) or to understand speech (receptive).

Apraxia The inability to carry out familiar and appropriate actions due to an apparent loss of memory of the sequences. There are two main types: *constructional*, where the person is unable to put together parts of an object to make a whole, and *motor*, where there is difficulty in performing a movement even though they understand the task.

Astereognosis An inability to identify objects by touch, in the absence of sensory loss.

Ataxia A disturbance of voluntary movement, seen as a marked lack of co-ordination of movement.

Attention A disturbance in the ability to attend for any period of time. This has a direct affect on the level of concentration.

Behavioural disturbances Any behaviour that manifests itself following the head injury and was not present before. It may be that behaviours are magnified, e.g. someone who was prone to losing their temper may now become violent, or there may be a totally new behaviour.

Body scheme/somatognosia A disturbance in body scheme involving a lack of awareness of body parts, an inability to name body parts and a lack of recognition of the relationship of body parts to each other.

Bradykinesia A slowness of movement.

Continence problems These may be incontinence of bladder, bowel or both. It is possible that catheterization will be necessary.

Dysarthria Refers to speech disturbances caused by a lack of muscular control of the speech organs.

Dyslexia Difficulty in reading and writing. This can appear with varying degrees of severity and may result in a total inability to comprehend written language.

Figure/ground discrimination Inability to distinguish by sight an object or figure from a competing background.

Hemiparesis/hemiplegia Lack of voluntary motor control affecting one side of the body.

Kinaesthetic awareness A loss of sensory input that can result in the inability to recognize objects by touch.

Laterality and directionality Inability to comprehend directions, such as right, left, up, down, etc.

Long- /short-term memory recall Inability to recall events that happened a long time ago or within a short space of time.

Loss of feeling A lack of sensory feedback that can result in loss of sensation of temperature and pain.

Physical/medical complications These may be fractures as a direct result of the accident or contractures that develop over time due to a lack of mobility.

Proprioception deficit A loss of feedback from surroundings present in many forms and may result in confusion and lack of orientation.

Quadriparesis/quadriplegia Inability to perform some or all voluntary movements in all four limbs can manifest itself with varying degrees of severity.

Spasticity Increase in muscle tone leads to stiffness and/or an inability to move limbs within the usual range.

Spatial orientation and awareness Inability to process information gained from surroundings. This can lead to severe confusion.

Tremor Tremor can be present in any part of the body, but is more common in head, trunk or upper limbs. It can severely restrict co-ordination.

Visual agnosia Failure to recognize an object through sight although vision is not impaired.

Visuo-spatial disorders Difficulty in recognizing the position of an object in space and its relationship to self or to another object.

One of the problems reported by those working with the head-injured is that there is no one person or discipline to treat the person. If we refer to the list of possible symptoms above, we see areas of expertise requiring a doctor, nurse, psychologist, speech therapist, physiotherapist, occupational therapist and/or social worker. Thus a wide variety of disciplines need to work with each individual, and the time span for this may be over a few years, making continuity difficult.

The types of problems that may occur during rehabilitation are often due to the cross-over of problems. If, for example, the person is referred to physiotherapy because they need specific help in regaining movements, the physiotherapist will look at the motor deficits of the person. If alongside this there are cognitive problems, i.e. the person is unable to understand what is being asked of them, has a poor short-term memory or has somatognosia, then the physiotherapist will find that their input is limited. If there is a behavioural problem, the person may refuse to co-operate. The same is true if they are referred to a speech therapist for help with aphasia or dysarthria; their work may be limited by cognitive problems as well as physical deficits.

Thus, to aid the rehabilitation process a detailed assessment must be done in order to prioritize the goals set. A complex programme of rehabilitation is required to ensure maximum benefit for the individual concerned.

There are many theories of learning, not detailed here, which, despite the differences between them, all agree on the importance of practice, feedback, goal specificity, and motivational and attentional variables (Fussey and Giles, 1988).

STAGES OF RECOVERY AND ASSESSMENT FOR REHABILITATION

Rehabilitation may take place in many forms and in a variety of settings. There are certain stages of recovery and rehabilitation.

- **Acute stage**
  This takes place within the hospital setting, and the initial stage will be while the person is still in a coma. They will need very special care at this stage to try to prevent secondary problems such as contractures, pressure sores, etc. In addition, active work will be done to try and rouse their level of consciousness. A number of professionals will be included, doctors, nurses and physiotherapists as well as the family.
- **Intermediate stage**
  This stage may still take place within the hospital setting following return to consciousness. The person may still require nursing staff but the rehabilitation process will also begin. Here we may see the input of a speech therapist, physiotherapist, psychologist etc. The results of this stage of rehabilitation will influence the next stage. A more detailed assessment of the neurological damage is possible at this stage.
- **Resettlement stage**
  This is defined by Wood and Eames (1989) as the move towards independence, and will involve a variety of professionals depending on the setting in which it takes place, perhaps a rehabilitation unit or at home. This will depend on the severity of the injuries and the type of rehabilitation process necessary for the individual.
- **Long-term recovery**
  Here we are looking at those individuals who will require long-term care and support. Again, this may take place in a variety of settings depending on the particular problems displayed by the person.

Throughout this whole period it is important that the individual is assessed regularly. There may be an initial conflict between being a 'patient' who is ill in hospital and moving towards being an active participant in their own rehabilitation. This conflict must be dealt with as it will hinder any further progress; a person cannot be a passive patient in a system of active rehabilitation.

Much support will be needed to make this transition for both the person and their family. Over time it is hoped that goals will be achieved. Priorities may also change, and if the rehabilitation is to be successful then this also needs to change according to the needs of the person. The priorities and expectations of both the individual and the family should be discussed and taken into consideration when developing the programme of rehabilitation.

One of the questions the individual and/or their families will want answered is that of the extent of the damage, the probability of recovery and the extent of recovery. In the early stages this is very difficult to answer as many of these factors are still unknown. As time goes on it will become evident where the greatest deficits lie. The long-term prognosis is very difficult as it will depend on the individual and their family as much as the rehabilitation service.

A guide was presented at the beginning of this chapter, however, any guide such as this must be used with caution. The individual will not want to hear that they cannot expect any further improvement, and the families will not want to accept that there can be no further improvement. However, realistic information must always be given, and if the rehabilitation programme is flexible and multidisciplinary, there will always be some room for improvement, no matter how slow, for the individual. It is the responsibility of the rehabilitation team to ensure that there is always a goal to work towards and that this is realistic and in line with the needs and priorities of the individual.

Thus, as time goes on from the onset of head injury, the goals will become more and more individualized, and the process of learning may be in ever smaller steps but can still take place. Rehabilitation is required from the initial accident throughout the life of the individual. If we look back at the incidence rate of 10% of one million per year, and that each person will require a rehabilitation programme that spans their life, then we are looking at a huge resource requirement, one which, in the majority of cases, cannot be met by the standard rehabilitation resources. It is, therefore, quite often up to the individual to seek further assistance when they have been discharged by the conventional system.

The time spent 'within the system' will depend on the severity of disability and the amount of care required and not necessarily on the individual's own expectations. It is at this stage, at present, that the conductor will meet the head-injured person.

THE CONSULTATION

As mentioned previously, in the United Kingdom, the conductor is more likely to come into contact with the severe head-injured person a few years after their accident. This is due, in part, to the rehabilitation service provided in this country and in part to the relatively new nature of this system here in the United Kingdom. As a result, the consultation will be very important to the conductor as it gives the opportunity to establish all the possible areas of neurological damage. Any programme set will, in its first stages, come from the information gained during this time.

APPLICATION FORM INFORMATION

Before the person attends they will have completed the basic application form described in Chapter 1. To this, further questions pertinent to individuals with head injury will have been added. Due to the diverse nature of head injury it is impossible to cover all areas of neurological damage, but some indicators can be given.

- date or year of accident
- length of time in coma
- presence of tremor, stiffness, loss of feeling
- contractures, noting the joints which are affected
- speech problems, type
- main method of communication
- memory problems, long- or short-term
- outline of present abilities during everyday activities, e.g. getting in and out of bed, dressing, washing, buttoning, main method of moving around, eating, drinking, bathing/showering, etc.
- continence problems, use of catheter
- receptive language skills
- regular drugs taken.

This information will give the conductor a clearer picture of the type of problems experienced by the person and an indication of the format required for the consultation. The person will be asked to bring any aids they use with them, such as communication or walking aids. This will allow the person access to the aids they use on a regular basis and will, in some cases, allow the conductor to communicate effectively with the individual.

ADDITIONAL INFORMATION

In the case of a head-injured person, medical reports will be essential. Progress reports from a rehabilitation programme will also be very useful. However, if there has been a long gap between rehabilitation and the conductive assessment, these may be difficult to obtain. If the person is still receiving therapy, then it is important that the conductor contacts the therapist concerned and receives an update on the work they are undergoing. It is also necessary for the individual concerned that the conductor works alongside other professionals and exchanges information with them on a regular basis.

During the consultation, the conductor needs to establish the priorities of the individual and to assess specifically what help can be offered through this system towards the achievement of these priorities. For this reason discussion during the consultation is important.

INFORMATION AT CONSULTATION

From the first introduction the conductor will obtain some information about the physical and communicative abilities of the person. These will give indicators to the following format. If the person displays greater physical deficit, then the conductor will have to perform a thorough assessment of motor abilities; if communication is a problem, the conductor may need to structure the consultation to establish the expressive and receptive language abilities of the person.

Due to the restriction of time and the setting of a consultation it would be impossible to make any concrete decisions following this. There are three main areas of development the conductor needs to observe: physical, cognitive, attention and behaviour.

Physical development

The conductor needs to see the person perform a few basic movements. These will enable the conductor to look for changes in muscle tone, ability to plan movements, ataxia, tremor and present range of movement. In addition, posture, balance and walking, if appropriate, can be observed. During discussion with the person, the conductor will have been able to establish the level of spontaneous movement as well as finer movements involved in speech, expression and gesture.

By asking the person to perform basic tasks, such as bending the right knee, the conductor will be able to see if there is a problem with body image. The extent of this may need to be explored further, but any problems of lateralization or somatognosia will become apparent. These must not be confused with problems related to receptive language, which will be more general throughout the consultation.

The conductor will assess the individual's ability to bend and stretch knees, the flexibility of hips, movements of extremities, i.e. hands, fingers, toes and ankles, the range of movement in all four limbs, the ability to change position by rolling to both sides, and sitting up. All these can be observed with the person in a lying position. This will ensure that the person feels secure.

If they have a high level of physical ability, the conductor may adapt these movements to be performed whilst sitting or standing. It is, however, very important that the person feels secure enough to produce the movements they are capable of, as this will prevent them from feeling that they have not been able to show all that they are capable of.

If a person finds it difficult to change position, then the conductor should not ask them to perform a whole string of more complex movements. The conductor is not aiming to find out what the person cannot do, but to establish their present level of ability. The conductor should help the person perform the movement, but only after allowing them the time they need, and must carefully observe and gauge when to step in and help.

Following basic movements, it may be pertinent for the conductor to ask the individual to perform more complex tasks, e.g. right heel on left knee, right hand on head, right foot flat, etc.

When the person is in a sitting position, the conductor will be able to observe finer hand movements and the general range of arm movements. Sitting posture and balance can also be observed. If necessary the person can sit in their own chair; this is particularly true if they find it difficult to balance in a sitting position.

If the conductor observes a lack of finer co-ordination, they may ask them to perform movements such as thumb on to nose to establish how accurate and precise these movements are.

There is no set physical routine the conductor uses to observe the individual. The consultation will be led by the abilities of the individual and therefore each assessment will vary.

Cognitive development

During discussion the conductor will have been able to observe for receptive aphasia, expressive aphasia, dysarthria and short- or long-term memory difficulties. It is very important that the whole assessment is directed to the individual and not to other members of the family. If they have difficulty speaking, then time must be given for them to express themselves as well as they can. If they use a communication aid then they should be given the opportunity to use this, as it will increase their independence and enable them to express their own wishes and not only the wishes of their family.

Attention and behaviour

In general a consultation will last about one hour, during which time the conductor will have been able to observe the ability of the person to attend. If there are any severe behavioural problems, it is likely that these will have emerged during the session.

The conductor needs to assess whether the person's needs would be best met within a group or in an individual session. The ability to attend, their level of concentration and their behaviour will be important factors in this process. If the person has a severe behavioural problem and is unable to co-operate, then it is likely that specialist help is needed. If their concentration span is short, it may be more beneficial if the individual works on a one-to-one basis with the conductor. If they are able to work with others, then a group session would be more appropriate.

In addition to the above, the conductor needs to ask specifically about loss of feeling, visual problems, continence problems, etc. There will have been some indication of problems in these areas on the application form, but the conductor may need to ask in more detail. This is particularly true if there are any problems with visual perception as these will have an effect on the way the programme is delivered.

Assessment of the head-injured person cannot take place in one hour alone, there may be more complex problems which become evident as the conductor begins working with the person. Continual progressive observation is essential for the conductor to gain a complete picture of the problems the individual faces.

PLANNING THE CONDUCTIVE PROGRAMME

As with other neurological problems, there are two levels of programme planning, **general** and **individual**. In the main, conductive education is carried out in groups, but there may be those who would benefit from individual sessions. Whether the person is a member of a group or whether they are in an individual session with the conductor, there will be aims for the group as a whole and for each individual. We will look specifically at a group programme; an individual programme will include the same aspects but will only cover the needs of one person rather than a whole group.

PLANNING A GROUP PROGRAMME

It may be appropriate for someone with a head injury to join a group with people with multiple sclerosis or those who have suffered a stroke. This would only happen if the conductor felt that their needs were more suited to another group. It is possible, for example, that a person with a head injury has ataxic symptoms similar to those of someone with multiple sclerosis, that they have hemiplegia like those who have had a stroke, or their problems may be similar to those of an adult with cerebral palsy.

The conductor, however, must exercise caution when placing someone in a group designed for those with a progressive disorder. If we are looking at rehabilitation following a head injury as following an upward curve, and rehabilitation of someone with a progressive disease as being maintenance, then there may be a conflict of interests between members of the group. The conductor needs to discuss this with all concerned in order to maintain a positive group atmosphere.

MULTIDISCIPLINARY AND INTERDISCIPLINARY APPROACHES

Bearing in mind that the person with a head injury is likely to have diverse needs, in many areas it has been suggested that a multidisciplinary approach is the most relevant (Garner, 1990). This can be taken one stage further where we have an interdisciplinary team and the forward planning is also done in a team.

The conductor is a professional in the area of neurological motor disorders, and the training for this encompasses all aspects of learning needed for a person with a motor disorder, including all cognitive problems, such as attention, motivation, aphasia, dysphasia and perception. Thus the conductive team consists of a team of professionals with a background in motor disorder.

All programmes, aims and goals will be set with the individual concerned and the team of conductors. This allows for an approach that provides continuity of expectations as well as continuity in performance (Russell and Cotton, 1994; Hári & Akos, 1988). As with any other team of professionals, the conductor team should review progress with the individual on a regular basis.

Thus the conductor, when planning the programme must take into consideration motor performance as well as deficits in cognition, communication and behaviour. Luria (Rosenthal *et al.*, 1990) identified four main principles of clinical work:

1. The principle of differential restoration of functional systems.
2. To take advantage of the intact cognitive processes.
3. Complete, extended programming of the restorative activity, i.e. tasks need to be broken down.
4. Constant signalization of the defect and effect of action, i.e. feedback.

PERSONALITY AND MOTIVATION

In Luria's earlier work he also recognized the influence of personality and motivation in the rehabilitative system. If we follow this as a guideline, then the conductor needs to take certain steps when developing a programme.

- The abilities of the individual are the starting point.
- All tasks must have a concrete goal, one which is meaningful and appropriate to the needs of the person.
- Tasks should be broken down into achievable components.
- Constant feedback should be given to enable the individual to evaluate their performance.
- The conductor must help to maintain interest level and motivation if the individual is to learn.
- Learning requires repetition; this must be in varying forms to distinguish between learning and habit.

The conductor will plan a programme from a basic task series as outlined in Chapter 12. This will provide the framework on which a programme can be built, but the programme should extend beyond the task series, and therefore it may be necessary for the carer and/or family to play an active part.

ELEMENTS SPECIFIC TO DIAGNOSIS

In addition to this basic programme specific elements must be built in which are tailor-made for one particular group. As mentioned previously some individuals may be better placed in a group of people with a different diagnosis, and the conductor would then follow the guidelines set out for that particular diagnosis. If the group is one created for individuals with head injury, the programme will need to be wide to encompass the varying problems.

It is impossible to give an outline for this as it would be too general. The following is an example of a possible mixed group taking part in a conductive education programme.

Example

Let us assume that there are six people in the group. The length of time since their accident varies from two years to six years. Two members are able to walk with the use of sticks or aids, two are able to walk alone for short distances and two are wheelchair users. Two members have a mild behaviour problem that makes it difficult for them to concentrate and co-operate for the whole session. One has receptive aphasia, another has expressive aphasia, two are ataxic, one is hemiplegic and the other three are quadriplegic. There are a variety of perceptual problems including body image and visual difficulties.

The conductor will have already assessed each of these people and will have individual goals for them.

Member 1
- to learn to increase weight-bearing on lower limbs when transferring
- to increase awareness of body image
- to reduce spasticity in all limbs
- to increase general range of movement
- to encourage active participation in everyday activities

Member 2
- to learn to bear weight through legs when standing
- to learn to transfer by standing
- to increase spontaneous movement in all limbs
- to encourage visual tracking of all movements

- to encourage verbal intention when performing the tasks

Member 3
- to learn to bear weight through legs when standing
- to encourage symmetrical posture
- to teach appropriate behaviour with other members of the group
- to encourage active participation within sessions
- to increase use of hands when performing everyday tasks

Member 4
- to teach how to fix limbs
- to learn appropriate direction of movements
- to increase awareness of body in space
- to improve balance in a standing position
- to learn to step whilst maintaining balance

Member 5
- to learn to maintain balance while walking on different surfaces
- to increase level of concentration
- to learn how to fix limbs in all positions
- to improve fluency of speech

Member 6
- to increase awareness of affected side
- to perform tasks from a mid-line position
- to learn to use arm as a support when performing spontaneous movements
- to link movements with speech, to verbalize the tasks

These aims will have been set in consultation with the individual and to help them to achieve the movements that are important for them.

The aims, whilst being specific, allow for many smaller stages. Any improvements must be immediately noted by the conductor and discussed with the person. It is very important to remember that the participant has a pre-morbid memory of their movements and therefore the improvements a conductor sees may not be noticed by them. Both the conductor and the individual are working from a different baseline, and the conductor must encourage the person each step of the way.

According to the composition of the group, the following general points will be included in the basic tasks series.

- The rhythm of the group must be slow to allow those with language and speech difficulties to participate fully.
- The verbalization of tasks should be short.
- A symmetrical, fixed position must be obtained before and following movement.
- Tasks should be varied to maintain attention.
- Tasks should be subdivided to allow for differences in physical ability, e.g. bend right knee – those who are able can then put right heel on left knee, then to the side, whilst those who need more time are bending their knee.

- Tasks should be performed in a lying, sitting and standing position. While some members are learning to bear weight on their lower limbs others may be walking.

In addition, the conductor will discuss with each individual how they are able to perform the task and which element of the task is of prime importance to them. It may be important for one person to reduce spasticity enough to be able to bend their leg, whilst someone else needs to be able to fix the movement. One member may be concentrating on the verbalizing of the tasks and another on understanding the task. This all happens simultaneously and it is the conductor's role to ensure that it does; if it does not, then the conductor needs to adapt the task series as necessary.

In order to meet any very specific needs the conductor may plan the programme to allow time for individual tasks. These may be in a sitting or standing position, and they may be cognitive, physical or communicative tasks. During this time the conductor must co-ordinate the group so that each member is active. The task set will include some element the person is able to do alone, together with the next stage where they will require assistance. Activities may be chosen where one member can assist another. There will be a combination of physical and verbal assistance provided, allowing everyone to remain active.

Depending on the ability of the group the conductor may wish to build more complex tasks into the basic tasks series.

Breathing tasks are very important for each member of the group since they can assist in reducing spasticity, increase fluency of speech, improve lung capacity, improve posture, and so on. These will be built into all programmes.

Basic positions, as referred to in the chapter on multiple sclerosis, will be the starting point for each movement. The conductor cannot think in terms of diagnosis only but in terms of needs; there will therefore be an overlap in the programmes for each diagnosis. The reader should refer to sections on programme planning in other chapters to gain an overall picture.

FACILITATION

There is no specific facilitation for the group of people with severe head injury. The conductor should follow the general guidelines for facilitation when working with each individual.

Facilitation used one day may not be the most appropriate for the following day. The most important facilitation for this group is to create an active working environment. It may be that the person is still trying to make the transition from being a patient to playing a role in their own rehabilitation. In order to achieve this the tasks set must be realistic and relevant. The person will need assistance to achieve their goal and yet must learn that they can achieve it alone. Conductive facilitation needs to be short term.

It is likely that participants will already be using various aids. These should be assessed regularly to ensure that they are still appropriate. This is usually done through the hospital, but the conductor needs to see that this assessment takes place. Unfortunately it is all too common that someone is using an aid that was needed following the accident, perhaps four years previously, that is now no longer beneficial. Communication aids may be used by those with severe speech problems, and these should be used alongside the tasks in the group.

Educational facilitation remains one of the most powerful aids with this group due to the diverse nature of their problems. Other types of facilitation should be used according to individual needs and the task set.

The reader should refer back to Chapter 1 to find which types of facilitation would be the most appropriate for each individual within the group.

SUMMARY

Severe head injury has many manifestations. Any number of problems may occur, in many variations, and the conductor needs to assess these as part of an ongoing process.

Goals set should be realistic, relevant to individual needs, and divided into logical stages if the participant is to play an active role.

Head injury, by its sudden nature, can have an enormous effect on the individual and the family. Help may be required in many directions and the conductor should be sensitive to the needs of all concerned.

Behaviourial and attention problems have an effect on the learning curve of the individual. If this is the case, then these should be a priority in rehabilitation. Varying educational techniques can be used to assist in this process.

The conductor usually meets with the individual some years following their accident, so they must maintain a realistic view of possible areas of improvement. This is particularly important with any system of rehabilitation that is new or outside our standard systems in the United Kingdom. The conductor must set realistic goals and explain these carefully to the individual and their family.

Conductive education cannot perform the impossible, but aims to build on the present abilities of the person in order to enhance learning. Learning may take place in small steps, but each small step will be another milestone for the individual concerned. The conductor's main role is to teach the person how to use their abilities, build on them and thus increase the role they can play in their everyday life. The areas of importance for this will be directed by the individual concerned and based on their personal wishes.

Stroke 10

This chapter outlines the main causes, types and manifestations of a stroke. Following this, it explores how conductive education can be applied to help individuals with this neurological condition.

The chapter includes:

- a brief outline of the causes and types of stroke
- an outline of the neurological damage caused by stroke
- the effects of a stroke on the abilities of the individual
- the consultation
- the planning of the conductive programme
- facilitation.

CAUSES AND TYPES OF STROKE

Stroke (Cerebral Vascular Accident) is the third commonest cause of death in the western world (Warlow, 1987). A stroke occurs suddenly, even though there may have been signs beforehand. It is a **very** traumatic incident. The person and their family may not have been aware of any signs and the stroke happens without any warning.

A stroke is caused either by a lack of blood to the brain due to a blockage of an artery, or by a rupture of an artery causing bleeding into or around the brain. There is a correlation between age and the incidence of stroke – it is rare under the age of 50 years, more common around 65 years, and the greatest risk is around the age of 80 years. There are five main causes.

- **Aneurysm**
  Ballooning of an artery. If this bursts, then there will be bleeding to the brain, causing the stroke.
- **Cerebral haemorrhage**
  Bleeding from an artery. It may be into the brain itself or into the

surrounding areas within the skull. This causes a severe stroke and accounts for about 15% of all cases.

- **Cerebral oedema**
  Swelling of the brain. The damage caused by this can be temporary if the pressure on the brain is reduced in time.
- **Cerebral infarction**
  Brain not receiving blood due to a blockage of an artery. This lack of blood is referred to as an **ischaemia**. If the blockage is not cleared within minutes, then this part of the brain will die. This is the commonest cause of stroke, accounting for about 80% of all cases.
- **Subarachnoid haemorrhage**
  Bleeding between the surface of the brain and the membrane. It is a common cause of stroke in young people, and in total accounts for about 5% of all cases.

NEUROLOGICAL DAMAGE CAUSED BY A STROKE

The effects of stroke will depend on the extent and nature of the areas damaged. The vast majority of human functions are controlled by the brain and therefore a variety of bodily or mental functions can be affected.

The motor area of the brain has nerve fibres which pass through the brain stem and into the spinal cord. These fibres are responsible for our voluntary movements. The fibres cross over where the brain stem meets the upper spinal cord, thus any damage to the right side of the brain affects voluntary movement on the left side and vice versa. This is known as the **pyramidal system**. It is therefore very important that the condition is defined specifically to avoid confusion.

Our voluntary movements are not only controlled in this way; there is another system known as the **extra-pyramidal system**. This is responsible for our automatic and unconscious movements. The fibres of this system run from the brain stem down to the spinal cord, therefore it is less likely that this system will be affected.

Loss of power caused by damage to the pyramidal system may vary from slight weakness to total paralysis. The variation will depend on the number of fibres affected by the stroke. Some functions may return when swelling has settled, but this is unknown at the time of the stroke.

RECOVERY AND REHABILITATION

Recovery from a stroke varies; in some cases it may be almost total, in others slight. The recovery that occurs spontaneously within the first few weeks can be quite rapid, following this, progress may be slower. There are varying schools of thought about how long recovery can take. Some feel that it can continue long term (Youngson, 1987), others see it as more short term, commenting that progress made after about six months will be almost negligible (Warlow, 1987). This will depend on how we view recovery.

The conductor will see recovery as a learning process, a relearning of skills applicable to the individual. If we accept that we all learn throughout our lives, then we can look at a long term recovery programme for the stroke survivor. The extent of function will depend on the damage caused, but learning and recovery are wider than physical function.

Rehabilitation is intensive following the stroke and during hospitalization, this will be gradually reduced over a period of 6 to 12 months. If the person wishes to continue to work towards their recovery following this, they are very often left to their own devices or the private sector. It is generally agreed that good management of this condition is essential in the early stages, however, longer term intervention is not typical, and thus the stroke survivor and their family are often left to seek their own help or accept the situation as it is.

EFFECTS OF STROKE ON ABILITIES

As mentioned previously, any number of functions can be affected by a stroke, and each individual will display different problems and to varying degrees. The following aims to outline the main effects possible following a stroke, however each case should be looked at individually. Certain patterns will be shown depending on the site of the stroke, and these too will be outlined.

LEFT-SIDE HAEMORRHAGE

Left-side haemorrhage affects the right side of the body. The following functions may be affected to some degree following a stroke on the left side of the brain.

Weakness or paralysis on right side

After time, this may develop into spasticity. It is common for the arm to be affected more than the leg. Any part of the body on this side can be affected, including the mouth and eye. It is possible that there may be a droop of the mouth to one side, which can cause dribbling or difficulty in eating.

There is a social implication to facial paralysis, since it is impossible for the person to smile in the way that they did before their stroke and they may appear more sombre.

Sensory loss

Sensory loss is very common and refers to a lack of feeling in some part of the body. If, for example this was on the sole of the foot, then the person would not know whether their foot was on the floor or not. This is very difficult for someone who has total feeling to understand, since it is one of those functions we know nothing about until we no longer have it. It can cause serious problems with regard to prevention of injury. This is particularly true if there is no feeling in the whole of a limb. For example if there is no feeling in the leg, then it is possible for the person to get it trapped underneath them when they are transferring. The same can be true of the arm. Any knocks or damage caused to a limb would not be felt, and therefore it is very important that limbs are checked regularly to ensure that there has been no injury or that there are no signs of cuts or sores. This applies also to judging temperature.

Very early in rehabilitation the person will need to learn how to compensate for sensory loss. In extreme cases the person may not be aware that the limb actually belongs to them because they have no feeling at all.

Aphasia
This is a disturbance in speech despite retaining the ability to articulate. There are two main types, expressive and receptive.

- **Expressive**
  Here the person is unable to say the correct word. In severe cases the person may be very fluent with speech but this speech will have no meaning for the listener. The stroke survivor will know exactly what they want to say, but the words will be incomprehensible to the listener.

  This is very frustrating for both parties and places an enormous strain on communication and relationships. In milder forms, a twenty questions game can be played until the correct word is found. Again, this can be time-consuming and frustrating for the carer as well as the stroke survivor.
- **Receptive**
  Here the person is unable to understand spoken language, which makes it very difficult for them to understand requests, conversation and media, such as television and radio. Language, which at one time was so natural, becomes a jumble of words with no meaning. In milder cases, the person will tend to answer inappropriately during conversations, or talk about subjects that are not related or relevant to the situation.

  In social situations they will tend to cut themselves off because they are unable to follow conversation. It is possible that all language becomes meaningless or that some words are difficult to comprehend.

  The severity of aphasia will depend on the extent of the damage caused by the stroke. The ability to relearn speech will depend on the nature and degree of the problem. Some recovery is to be expected, but this may be limited in some cases.

These two forms do not always occur in their pure form, it is possible to see a mixed form in some individuals. Intensive rehabilitation is needed for any one who has aphasia.

Dyslexia
The ability to read the written word is affected. The letters and words have no meaning, even though the person can see them clearly.
Dysphagia
This is a difficulty in swallowing and can affect eating, as the person may find it difficult to swallow food. Chewing is not necessarily affected. It also tends to cause excessive salivation and dribbling because the person is unable to automatically swallow the saliva formed in the mouth. This has social implications for them when in company.
Dyscalculia
Dyscalculia is an impairment in numerical ability that may include the understanding of numerical values and/or ability to perform any form of mathematical problem. This can have social implications in the handling of money.
Visual problems
The most common problem is the loss of field of vision on the affected side. This is called **hemianopia**. The eyes move in all directions but each eye will only process half the information within the field of vision. In severe cases a person may eat only half of the food on their plate and not realize that the other half is there. As this will always apply to the affected side, vision of the affected limbs is restricted. This, together with a possible sensory loss, means that the person can lose all concept of that side of their body.

Generally, we rely on two main types of feedback for an awareness of the position and presence of our limbs: visual and sensory. Without these we have no concept of that part of our body and this can lead to difficulties with rehabilitation.

RIGHT-SIDE HAEMORRHAGE

Right-side haemorrhage affects the left side of the body. The following functions may be affected to some degree after a stroke on this side of the brain.
Weakness or paralysis of the left side
This can include any part of the body, to a degree that will vary between individuals. After a time the paralysis may develop into spasticity. As with a left-side haemorrhage, the arm tends to be more affected than the leg.
Loss of visual memory
The person is unable to recognize objects from past experience. They may know the word for an object but will be unable to connect this with the visual form of that object. It is possible that they will not recognize people or places. This can be very disturbing for the family as it is possible that loved ones will not be recognized and home will be a new experience for the person. If there are no other memory or language problems, the person is able to relearn.

Psychological effects

These effects can include mood swings, sudden emotional upset for no apparent reason, a sense of hopelessness and a lack of confidence. It is possible that in severe cases the person may change their personality completely.

This is very difficult for the family to cope with, as the person following the stroke may be very different from the one they loved before the stroke. The family can become very despondent and frustrated and will need a lot of support to cope with their own feelings. It is very important that relatives understand the problem as this often helps them to support their loved ones.

Shortening of attention span

This is very characteristic of people who have suffered a stroke affecting their left side. The person may be unable to concentrate for more than a few minutes and this can affect their ability to follow a conversation, concentrate on their movements, watch television programmes, read a book, etc. The person will become very restless as they are unable to fill their time, and they will need many activities in order to prevent them from becoming frustrated.

Loss of memory

Loss of long-term memory makes it very difficult for the person to relate to events that happened before the stroke. Conversation tends to revolve around the stroke, hospitals, and so on. This is not necessarily because they only have a memory of recent events, but may also be due to the fact that this is the most relevant subject for them at this time. This improves when the person leaves hospital and is able to increase their experience.

Loss of short-term memory can be temporary or permanent. If permanent, then the carer needs a great deal of support since the person cannot usually be left on their own. They may not know that they have eaten, they may not know where they live if they go out; they may go to the kitchen and not remember why they went. A short-term memory problem can impede progress in rehabilitation since they are unable to build on each stage of learning.

Depression

This depression is different to the feeling of despair following a natural traumatic event that is likely to improve with support and help. Depression caused by the damage to the brain needs medical treatment in order to control it. The family will also need support in order to understand and cope with the problem.

Dysarthria

Here the formation and articulation of words will be affected although the linguistic ability remains intact. The listener may have difficulty understanding what is said as speech may not be very clear.

Visual problems

As with a left-side haemorrhage, there can be a loss of visual field with a right-side haemorrhage as well.

Neglect of affected side

This neglect can be in the form of a denial, where the person does not believe that the limbs belong to them. In severe cases they may actually be disturbed by the presence of this limb, as it does not belong to them, but they are unsure who it belongs to. In milder forms, the person will find it very difficult to build up a body image that includes the left side, as it is no longer automatic to include it as a part of their body. This is separate from the physical problems of lack of movement.

The limb or limbs may appear ugly to them, in the way, and they may hate the fact that they are there. Families will naturally encourage the person to be aware of the affected side and try to convince them that it is a part of them, but the person can continually insist that it is not theirs. If the families do not understand that this is the result of brain damage, they tend to assume that there is intellectual damage, because it is hard for them to imagine that a person can deny a part of their body.

BRAIN STEM STROKE

This can affect **all** movements of the body parts except the eyelids. Functions such as hearing, vision, memory and intellect remain intact. This is often referred to as the **locked in** syndrome, because the person is locked within their own body. Other specific functions that may be affected include:

- movement of the eyes in any direction
- problems with swallowing
- articulation difficulties making speech difficult
- balance
- breathing can become very shallow
- weakness on both sides, the extent of which will depend on the severity of the stroke
- double vision.

We can see from the above that a wide variety of functions, including movement, speech, understanding, sensation, psychological function or vision can be affected as a result of a stroke.

Although there will be certain characteristics depending on the area of damage, it is impossible to discover which functions will be affected and to what extent. This makes it very difficult for the families, as this is the first question they ask when the person has suffered the stroke. The answer to this question is, therefore, usually a little vague, because there is no way of being specific until the person has begun to make some recovery.

It is very important that the families are informed of the manifestations as they become clear to the medical staff. Alongside this, an explanation of longer term effects and the rehabilitation process should also be shared with them as soon as possible.

THE CONSULTATION

The conductor, from training and experience, must have a good working knowledge of the effects of a stroke. This will give a good baseline from which to assess the individual manifestations relevant to the person attending for consultation. The consultation serves to enable each individual to discuss their priorities and goals for rehabilitation, and for the conductor to assess if help can be given in these areas, what form it should take and to explain the system of conductive education. The consultation will then be followed up in writing.

It is very important that there is a two-way communication during the consultation. If the person has difficulty speaking, then time must be given to allow them to communicate. If a communication aid is used, this should be brought along to the consultation to ensure maximum communication between the conductor and the applicant. It is very common for the carer and/or family member to answer questions for the person if they have difficulty speaking. The conductor should encourage the person to communicate but may need to include the carer in the conversation. The conductor must be careful not to exclude the person and talk only to the carer, this lowers self-esteem and only enables the conductor to find out the priorities of the carer and not necessarily of the person concerned.

APPLICATION FORM INFORMATION

Before attending for consultation the person will have completed an application form. This will include the information described in Chapter 1 together with more specific information required for people who have suffered strokes, such as:

- which side of the body is affected and to what degree, i.e. paralysis, spasticity
- presence of sensory loss, to what degree and on which part of the body
- presence of aphasia and difficulties incurred
- main method of communication, if relevant
- presence of contractures, in which part of the body
- breathing capacity, any reduction since stroke
- level of concentration
- depression, length of bouts
- presence of memory problems, details including short- or long-term memory.

- swallowing ability
- continence of bowels and bladder
- any drugs taken regularly, any known side-effects.

In addition to this, it is very important to gain information from the person's general practitioner regarding blood pressure levels. It is quite common for stroke sufferers to have high blood pressure and this should be known before they undertake any form of physical exertion. If this blood pressure is not under medical control then it is likely that the person would not be fit enough to take part in the conductive programme. Information is also required about the heart, diabetes, epilepsy and if there has been any other serious illness.

With the above information in mind, the conductor is able to structure the consultation to discover the severity of the condition and the practical implication of any neurological deficits. Each individual will differ with regard to the effect of their stroke, their ability to manage their condition and their priorities for rehabilitation. The conductor needs this information to help create an overall picture to enable them to set realistic goals for the person.

INFORMATION AT CONSULTATION

From first meeting, the conductor will be able to observe spontaneous movements, speech, gesture, understanding, ability to walk, balance, taking coat off, etc. This information is as important as the formal information gained during the consultation. It is possible for a stroke survivor to relearn specific movements, but these may be isolated and not applied in spontaneous situations.

During initial discussion with the person about the information on the application form, the conductor will have had the opportunity to look at the degree of spontaneous movement of the affected limbs. In addition, the level of verbal communication, understanding of speech, extent of facial paralysis and, to some degree, the level of neglect on the affected side will have been observed.

It is very important that the conductor creates an informal atmosphere to allow the person to feel as comfortable and as relaxed as possible. The conductor must not forget that they will be very nervous, very unsure of what to expect, and it is up to the conductor to ease this pressure and thus allow them to show their full potential.

If appropriate, the conductor will then ask the person to write their name and a short sentence. This will help to show up any other deficits, such as dyslexia. If the person is unable to write due to the physical effect of the stroke, then the conductor should not ask them to do this task.

Basic movements

The conductor will then ask the person to perform a few basic movements, which will help to indicate the physical capabilities of the person, their ability to understand simple commands, their body image and understanding of body parts.

Basic movements, such as transferring from sitting to lying, rolling to one side and then the other, bending knees, lifting legs, lifting arms up, will be performed. The specific nature and type of movement requested will depend on the individual's baseline abilities. The conductor should give them the opportunity to show the movements they are able to do and not only look for the ones that they cannot.

During all these movements, the conductor will ask the person to do only what they can. Once they have done this, the conductor can help them so they achieve the movement. If they have little spontaneous movement, then the conductor must immediately find a way for them to perform some movements successfully. For example they may clasp their hands and lift their clasp up to chest height.

It is very important that the person does not over-perform movements and disregard any pain that this may incur. This is particularly relevant if the person has a subluxated shoulder. In this instance the conductor needs to ascertain the degree of movement without causing pain. In the wish to perform well, many applicants are reluctant to say if movements are painful, also there may be a lack of feeling which prevents them feeling pain. The conductor must observe facial expression and expression of the eyes in order to ensure that the person is not in pain.

Following movements in a lying position, the person will be asked to sit up and, if possible, sit alone on the edge of the bed or plinth. If they need support when sitting, the person can transfer into their chair where they feel secure. Throughout all these movements the conductor will have been observing the range of movement with the affected limbs, overall co-ordination of movements, how much the person compensates for the affected side, any sign of neglect of the affected side, lateralization problems, tolerance to physical movements, concentration and visual abilities.

In a sitting position the conductor will also ask the person to lift and bend their legs, move their ankles and toes if possible, as well as performing arm and hand movements. The conductor can observe their ability to balance, their awareness of the affected side as well as specific physical capabilities.

Cognitive abilities

In addition to observing physical movements, the conductor needs to establish the cognitive abilities of the person. It is important that understanding of language, of the written word, numbers, the concept of shape, lateralization, visual neglect, memory capacity and any other problem areas are assessed. In order to do this, the conductor may set specific tasks for the individual. These will have been prepared in advance using the information from the application form together with the conductor's knowledge of the condition and possible ways of testing cognitive abilities.

GOALS AND PROVISION

By this stage in the consultation, the conductor should have a clear picture of the person's capabilities, their priorities and their cognitive abilities. Specific questions may be asked if the conductor requires further clarification on their observations.

The conductor will then ascertain how conductive education could help the person and the type of provision that would enable goals to be reached. These goals must be discussed immediately with the person and should be set from as broad a knowledge of the person as possible. It is important that a positive but realistic overview of the observations is shared with both the person and their carer, thus giving the person the opportunity to discuss this and ask any further questions. They will then have some time to consider the proposals set during the consultation and the recommendations for placement. In some cases individual sessions may be appropriate. This will depend on the individual concerned, the severity of their condition and their ability to participate in group activities.

The information gained at consultation provides the basis for the programme the person will follow. It is important, however, that this programme is carefully monitored because the conductor will only have seen the person for a short time and in a formal setting.

PLANNING THE CONDUCTIVE PROGRAMME

There are two main levels of programme planning – **general** and **individual**. The conductor will have a basic programme designed to teach people who have suffered strokes. A basic structure of tasks as outlined in Chapter 12 would be the starting place for each group. The conductor does not need to write a completely new programme each time a person joins an established group. The group programme would need to be adapted slightly to incorporate the aims relevant for that person, but the overall programme would remain the same.

The following programme planning material assumes that the conductor is establishing a new group for people who have suffered strokes. Once this is established, the programme would only adjust for a new group member.

From the basic task series, the conductor will build up or break down tasks as appropriate for the group or individual. It is very important that all relevant functions are covered in the task series, and that learning is broad-based and not a narrow-based motor programme. The programme may need to be gradually built up over time, and new elements introduced as the group make progress.

OVERALL AIMS FOR STROKE SUFFERERS

Neurological damage caused by a stroke is not progressive, thus the conductor will need to prioritize the goals for each individual in the group. This will have been done for each person during their consultation. The goals for each individual are then built into the group programme.

Conductive education for the stroke survivor has the main aim of teaching skills that are applicable in everyday life and not taught in a functional way that would inhibit transference of personalized skills. Each person will have their own way of performing movements. There is no prescription for getting out of a car, sitting on a chair or washing the dishes, each person will do these in their own way, depending on ability and past experience. Conductive education aims to teach the person the **components** of everyday skills that they can apply to their own situation. Once these skills are put together and applied, then learning has taken place.

Certain structured activities may play a part within the programme, for example peeling vegetables, washing up, making tea and coffee. These serve as teaching sessions for the conductor to show the person how to apply skills learnt within the session, thus giving the person a base on which to build.

PREVENTION OF CONTRACTURES

It is very important following a stroke, especially in the early stages, that the person does not develop contractures. Full range of movement must be maintained in order to assist the person to achieve their goals.

At first it may be that the priority for the person is to learn how to balance in a standing position; hand movements may seem less important. However, if the conductor concentrated on one function only, then the potential for rehabilitation would be reduced. It may take some time for the person to learn to stand, and their next priority may be to walk. Again, more time is needed, and if throughout this period the hand has been neglected because it is not a priority, then it is likely that contractures of the wrist and shoulder will have begun to form.

If the person then sees hand movement as their next priority, those movements will be restricted due to the contracture, thus they will not achieve the movements that may have been possible immediately following the stroke. The programme should therefore be balanced to include all movements, as well as prioritizing goals for each member.

APHASIA

If the person has aphasia then the programme must be designed to increase their receptive or expressive language skills. It is possible that verbal instructions will have to be broken down to allow active participation. One or two significant words may be chosen from the instruction.

Example

If the task is to put the right foot flat, the verbal intention would be **I put my right foot flat**. A person with a language difficulty would not be able to participate fully in this, so the conductor would break down the verbal intention. The method of doing this will depend on the main problem shown by the person.

If they had a lateralization problem, the intention may become **right foot**; if they had severe problems naming body parts, then the intention may be **foot**; if they had difficulty with spacial awareness then it may be **foot flat**. The conductor should use the information gained at consultation and the overall aims of the whole group to establish the best verbal intention for each group.

As the person begins to learn, the conductor builds up the verbal intention. If they are receiving speech therapy, then it would be advisable for the conductor to meet with the speech and language therapist in order to maintain continuity for the individual.

COGNITIVE, SOCIAL AND PSYCHOLOGICAL FUNCTIONS

Tasks do not only relate to speech and movement functions, although these may play a large role. Other functions, such as cognitive, social and psychological, must also be built into the whole programme. Specific activities may be included for this, or time may be allowed at the end of the session for the members to talk and have coffee, thus giving them the opportunity to apply the skills they have been learning into a practical situation that enhances their learning.

The group can have a strong effect on the individual, and it is important that the conductor guides the group towards a positive learning environment. It is very easy for individuals to sit and compare notes on their difficulties and, although this is very important, the solution should be the priority. The conductor needs to help the group to share their experiences in a positive way, as this is also an important element of the overall programme in conductive education.

All tasks carried out need to be performed both with the affected and non-affected side, enabling the person to gain an internal picture of the movement that will help to improve overall body image and co-ordination as well as preventing dependency on the unaffected side, and denial of the affected side.

During the days, months and years following a stroke, the person will endeavour to adapt their movements to enable the non-affected side to compensate for the affected one. This is a very natural short-term solution. However, in the long term, it may create problems as the person will be unable to maintain a central position. Gradually the centre of gravity moves over to the non-affected side and overall co-ordination can be affected. As the centre of gravity moves it becomes increasingly difficult to transfer weight from one foot to the other, thus balance and walking are difficult. Activities such as putting a coat on can become difficult because the person is unable to balance securely. Thus it is very important that the conductor helps the person to maintain a mid-line position, and the affected side is incorporated as much as possible into their everyday activities.

COMMON ELEMENTS

As discussed above, the conductor will structure the programme to suit the needs of each group. There will, however, be some common elements that can be built into all groups of stroke survivors.

- All movements should be started from a central position whether this is when lying, sitting or standing.
- All movements should be confirmed with visual feedback, i.e. the person should always look at their limbs when moving them. Naturally this is not relevant in a standing position, but if done when sitting and lying then they will be aware of the position of their limbs when standing and have increased security.
- Movements with clasped hands assist in an active way movements of the affected hand. They also help to promote a mid-line position.
- All movements should be verbally intended to improve language skills, increase concentration and awareness of movements.
- The rhythm for each group should be relatively slow to allow time to reduce spasticity and perform a relaxed movement.
- All movements should be carried out with the affected limb, non-affected limb and both together.
- Constant feedback of the position of the affected limb must be given by the conductor.
- All movements should be carried out within the maximum possible range of movement.

In addition to the task series described above, the conductor may build in other common elements to the programme. These could include:

- construction of objects following verbal or written instructions
- specific work on breathing and articulation
- sequencing of events
- naming of objects
- naming of colours
- relearning sequences, such as days of the week, months of the year
- reading, comprehending and identifying with written material.

These elements will depend on the major areas of damage from the stroke, the level of rehabilitation previously received and the level of the person at the time of attendance.

CONSISTENCY

As with all neurological conditions, consistency in approach is vital to the stroke survivor. During their stay in hospital and subsequent rehabilitation it is likely that they will have encountered a whole team of therapists and doctors. Many efforts are made to ensure that the approach to the individual is consistent, but this is very difficult when rehabilitation covers so many disciplines over a prolonged period of time.

Kinsman (1987) suggests one of the possible reasons for the breakdown in a team is that each member works within their own role or discipline and has their own goal for the person. This may present difficulties in sharing goals across different disciplines: a physiotherapist may be working towards increased mobility; a speech therapist towards improving articulation; and an occupational therapist to improving ability to take part in dressing and washing. These goals are functionally based and therefore it is very difficult to find a common thread between them.

Kinsman also highlights the problem of time lapse between assessment of the person and the setting of common goals. The conductor, as a specialist in the area of neurological motor disorder, is able to set goals across the range of functions, thus making continuity easier to maintain. The approach remains the same whether cognitive, physical or verbal functions are being addressed. This ensures a good, positive learning environment that promotes learning.

ACTIVE PARTICIPATION

The active participation of the individual in the process of setting goals, assessing priorities and carrying out the programme all assist in giving the person control over their own rehabilitation and seeing that they play a part in achieving this. This helps general well-being as well as increasing motivation, confidence and learning.

The inclusion of prime carers, families and other relevant professionals is of great importance. The family need to be given guidance so that they too can play a role in the rehabilitation process. Very often they adopt a role similar to that of the nurse in the hospital because their role has never been defined or discussed with them. If the carer is given a specific role in supporting the individual, then they too are able to help in the process. For many families it may be their first experience of disability, and they will not have the knowledge and experience of the professional. It is therefore up to the professional to share their expertise with the families.

The conductive group should include participants with a variety of problems. This allows them to learn from each other and experience success. If there are members who have speech difficulties, then it is important that they work alongside others who have speech. This not only provides them with a language-enriched environment, but they can learn from others in a similar situation. This is very important, since a conductor or any other professional is unable to place themselves totally in the situation of the stroke survivor, and the support they receive from each other cannot be matched by a professional.

The conductor has a responsibility to set out the programme tasks, observe the participants' progress and lead the group. They must also facilitate each individual so that they achieve success and learn how to perform the movements they require.

FACILITATION

As with all other conditions, facilitation should include educational and mechanical forms of facilitation as described in Chapter 1.

The stroke survivor is in a unique position in that one side of the body functions well. This can be both an advantage and a disadvantage. They are able to compensate for some of the loss of function by using the non-affected side and they are also able to use this side to assist the affected one, however, it is very important that they do not learn to over-compensate and continue using the non-affected side as an aid instead of a replacement.

There are two main ways this can be achieved.

- When moving with the non-affected side, they should try to be aware of **how** they have performed the movement, and register the feeling and the involvement of other parts of the body. This can then be replicated when performing movements with the affected side, and it is often helpful when trying to initiate a movement.
- The person uses the non-affected side to directly assist the affected side in a way that promotes active movement. An example of this would be

clasping hands. This enables the person to move their affected arm and hand but still receive feedback from the active movement. This is very different from a passive movement because the person has initiated the movement themselves. It is not enough to just clasp hands, they must also try and increase the role of the affected hand. By performing movements in this way the person is able to achieve success whilst building up the active movements of the affected arm.

For these methods to be used successfully, the person must know why they are performing movements in this way; they must know what they are trying to do. It is the conductor's role to explain this to them and show them the technique for achieving this. Manual assistance by the conductor may be necessary in the early stages, but this should be minimal and reduced as soon as possible to promote active participation.

VISUAL AND VERBAL FEEDBACK

Visual and verbal feedback play an important role especially if there is loss of sensation without this the person will be unaware of the movements they are producing. In a lying position they should be given a box or pillow to rest the head on so that they can see their movements without having to lift their head or hold their head in mid-air. In this position they can begin to register their movements and increase their body awareness.

When sitting, the person is able to glance down at their lower limbs in order to receive feedback; it is, however, impossible for them to see their upper body and monitor their posture if there is loss of sensation. Mirrors are very helpful in this situation, but it can be confusing to adjust your position according to a mirror image. The conductor, therefore, must provide verbal feedback and correction for each individual. In this way they will begin to learn how to maintain their posture and increase the awareness of their limbs. If they are standing and have to move their head to see the position of their lower limbs, then their balance point will alter and make their standing position not only insecure but difficult to monitor.

Verbal feedback from both the conductor and the family is very important for the individual but it must be controlled. The person is likely to require a great deal of intervention in the early stages, and if they are constantly being corrected then they will become very despondent. Therefore the correction given must be relevant to the individual's personality and the conductor should discuss this with them and their close family in order to find a suitable level.

RHYTHMICAL INTENTION

Rhythmical intention plays an important part in the system of conductive education. This is described in detail in Chapters 4 and 5.

We know that it is very important that the appropriate verbal intention is given in accordance with any language difficulties. In addition to this, the appropriate rhythm for each group must be found. As a general rule the more severe the spasticity the slower the rhythm.

For the person to perform a meaningful movement they must learn to do it in a relaxed way; any sudden change in position will increase the spasticity and the result will be counter-productive. They need to learn how to move without increasing spasticity, and also how to control their upper limb whilst moving the lower limb to prevent simultaneous movements. When they are able to perform a relaxed movement, the rhythm can increase a little in tempo. This is one of the most difficult skills for the individual to learn, so the conductor must give the knowledge, assistance and support to achieve it.

ADAPTING THE TASKS

The breaking down and building up of tasks is very important as it enables each person in the group to work at their own level whilst still having a role as a member of the group. If the task is to roll on to the left side, some individuals may hold on to a chair and pull themselves over, others may use their right leg to help push themselves over, some may perform this with clasped hands to prevent the affected arm becoming trapped and others may be able to perform this alone. Each individual must find their own solution.

The breaking down of tasks also assists with language difficulties. Even if the person is physically capable of producing a complex movement, this does not mean that they will always be required to do so. The task may be to put right heel on left knee and right hand on left shoulder. This instruction may be too complex for them to understand even though they are physically capable of performing it. In this situation the conductor must be aware of all the needs of the person and not just motor needs. The task should be broken down into components to assist with execution, and as they learn the instructions so it can be built up.

In order to ensure learning, the conductor must vary the task series at times. If the person always completes the same tasks in the same order then it will be unclear whether learning has taken place or whether habits are forming. Again this is very important with regard to receptive aphasia. It is beneficial to the person to follow a structured programme at first as this will give them confidence. The conductor needs to determine when this can be changed. It may be that instead of starting with the right leg, the conductor asks the person to start with the left leg, as this will give an indication of whether lateralization has improved. In doing this, however, the conductor must be aware of the need to maintain the overall structure of the programme – any changes to the order must not subtract from the structure of tasks.

MECHANICAL FACILITATION

Mechanical facilitation can play a role with stroke survivors. The following are some examples that may be incorporated, depending on the severity of the participants' condition. They must be seen as facilitators of movement.

- Lift the wrist up and the fingers will automatically stretch; push the wrist down and the fingers will bend. This can be used in the teaching of grasp and release. The person needs to learn how to move their wrist as this helps to regain function in the fingers.
- Place the back of the hand on a table, relax it and the fingers will begin to open.
- Extend the thumb away from the palm then the palm will stretch. Here the person is able to use their non-affected hand to help with the affected one.
- Roll on to one side, relax the top leg over the edge of the bed and the knee will begin to bend. This can be used to assist with bending the knee. The individual is able to learn how to actively use their hips to initiate flexion of the knee.

It is important to remember that **no mechanical facilitation is better then mechanical facilitation**, so the conductor should only use mechanical facilitation when necessary.

Rhythmical intention can be learnt by the individual and applied throughout their day, and educational facilitation is the basis of group work for the conductor. Facilitation must be varied to remain meaningful. The individual must not become dependent on facilitation from the conductor since this will prevent them from transferring the skills they have learnt into their own home. The conductor should gradually decrease their assistance, and in this way the person is able to learn and achieve success.

SUMMARY

The main principles of conductive education apply to all neurological conditions and this chapter should not be read in isolation. It outlines the specific elements the conductor must consider when working with stroke survivors, but experience of other conditions can also help.

Conductive education aims to help the stroke survivor increase awareness and the level of voluntary movement on the affected side. All other functions must be taken into consideration since the damage caused by a stroke can be wide and varied. Each individual must be taken on their own merits and the conductor must establish a good working relationship with them based on mutual trust.

The conductor must work alongside other professionals if the individual is receiving services from others. This is very important for the individual and will increase their rate of progress.

Families and carers should also be considered. The conductor needs to discuss their role with them and guide them towards taking an active part in rehabilitation. They must not feel excluded, neither should they feel that the success of any rehabilitation is dependent wholly on them. The conductor must respect the priorities of both the individual and the carer, which may be very different.

Underlying the whole of conductive education is the knowledge that the conductor is working with adults who have past experiences, individual personalities and lifestyles and who are aware of their needs in rehabilitation. In turn the conductor can provide the expertise to assist the person in finding the route towards achieving the goals that are important to them.

Cerebral palsy in adulthood

11

This chapter outlines the neurological conditions classed as cerebral palsy, and the manifestations of these conditions in adulthood. Cerebral palsy is a non-progressive childhood disorder, but we often forget that the children of today will be the adults of tomorrow.

The adult with cerebral palsy may present a different picture to the child and it is the intention here to focus on the adult and the implications for them of congenital neurological deficits. For this purpose school leavers will be referred to as adults, and the scope of the chapter thus extended to cover adolescence as well as adulthood.

Conductive education in the United Kingdom began with children with cerebral palsy. Many think that the system only applies to these children, but conductive education, as a system of rehabilitation, in fact has its roots with adults and therefore has significance in the field of adult cerebral palsy. The needs of this client group will, however, be very different, and will have to be met in an appropriate way.

The chapter includes:

- a brief summary of cerebral palsy
- manifestations of neurological damage and implications for adults
- the consultation
- the planning of the conductive programme
- facilitation.

TYPES OF CEREBRAL PALSY

By definition cerebral palsy is a non-progressive neurological disorder occurring in young children. The impairment in motor function may be in the form of paresis, involuntary movement or inco-ordination. Alongside motor function, other functions may also be damaged. The location in the brain, of the damage, will determine the form and degree of the impairment and whether other neurological functions are also impaired.

Cerebral palsy is the result of some form of trauma between conception and early childhood. There are five main periods when the unborn foetus or the small baby can be at risk.

1. Prenatal – greatest risk between 13 and 25 weeks
2. Premature delivery – deliveries between 26 and 36 weeks
3. Perinatal – trauma during labour or delivery
4. Neonatal – up to around 28 days
5. Postnatal – from one month; this however accounts for a small percentage of children who have cerebral palsy.

SOURCE OF DAMAGE

In order to understand the differing types of cerebral palsy, it is necessary to look at the source of the damage, the brain. There are three main areas of the brain identified as playing a role in the control of movement and posture. Cerebral palsy refers to damage in any of these areas, but in order to be more specific we must look at the roles of these areas.

The three areas are the motor cortex, basal ganglia and cerebellum, and damage in any of these areas will produce a range of symptoms.

Motor cortex

The cells in the motor cortex are responsible for our conscious, voluntary movements. The cells on one side of the brain control movements on the opposite side of the body. These cells are linked, by axons, to the spinal cord. Damage along the axon or within the cell body itself will impair functions. This takes the form of **spasticity**. The extent and nature of the damage will vary according to its site. It is possible that damage is on one side of the body only, **spastic hemiplegia**, or that the legs only are affected, **spastic diplegia**. If all four limbs are affected, then the term **spastic quadriplegia/tetraplegia** is applied.

Basal ganglia

The motor pathways mentioned above are insufficient to control our movements completely. The basal ganglia has a function in our posture and tone. This helps us to use gravity to its maximum to find positions in line with gravity, using minimal strength. Any damage to this area will produce flailing, jerky movements, immobility or stiffness (**athetosis** or **dystonia**).

Cerebellum

The main role of the cerebellum is the co-ordination of our actions together with balance. Any damage to this area will result in a lack of co-ordination, shakiness and a general unsteadiness of movement, **ataxia** which usually affects all four limbs.

Cerebral palsy can manifest itself in any of the above ways depending on the area of the brain damaged. The extent of the disability is directly related to the damage. Usually the clinical picture is more complicated than suggested above. Damage is rarely limited to one single area of the brain, therefore we usually see symptoms which affect intellect, vision, hearing, etc. Cerebral palsy is not, in all cases, linked purely to movement disorders, but there are a large number of associated disabilities. These will be discussed in detail in the next section.

Damage to the areas of the brain outlined above do not only occur with cerebral palsy but can also result from acquired disorders such as head injury, stroke and Parkinson's disease. There will therefore be an overlap in the symptoms between these conditions. The effect of the neurological damage should be considered rather than just its location. The implications of the neurological damage will be individual, the person and how it affects them is of central importance. There will also be a natural overlap in the rehabilitation or habilitation of adults with motor disorders.

FROM CHILDHOOD TO ADULTHOOD

By the onset of adulthood the cerebral palsied child will have undergone some form of education and habilitation. This may have taken place in the home, school or residential care setting. The specific type of cerebral palsy diagnosed often gives an indication to the independence of the young person.

Soboloff in Stanton (1992), performed a study of young adults over the age of 20 years diagnosed with spastic diplegia and spastic hemiplegia. Of these, 48% were self-sufficient, 30% received part-time care, 22% received total care and 31% were in full time employment. These figures, however, do not include other, more severe forms of cerebral palsy. In addition Bleck (1987) reported that cerebral palsied adults aged above 18 years were more likely to have serious emotional breakdowns than those under 18 years. This gives an indicator to the changing manifestations of the condition, despite it reportedly being a non-progressive disorder.

Unfortunately, reality often strikes once a child leaves school, particularly if the child has been a high achiever. The cold reality is that society is not a friendly place for a disabled adult. Views may have begun to change over the years but there is still a long way to go. Whilst we are, as a society, more tolerant of the young disabled child, our tolerance decreases as the young person ages.

NEUROLOGICAL DAMAGE AND ITS IMPLICATIONS IN ADULTHOOD

In this section the symptoms of cerebral palsy as they manifest themselves in adulthood are examined. As mentioned previously, cerebral palsy is a non-progressive neurological condition where the implications of the symptoms change as the young person ages. This can be due to a number of factors, including orthopaedic, social and emotional. There will also be an enormous variation in the degree and number of symptoms shown.

CEREBRAL PALSY IN ADOLESCENCE

Without looking into the details of the cerebral palsied child, it is important to mention that any child with a movement disorder will have less access to their surroundings, and this can affect their ability to learn through experience. They may be unable to join in all activities with their peer group and this will naturally disadvantage them socially.

When reaching adolescence the young person is likely to become increasingly aware of their body and its limitations. This can cause emotional confusion and in some instances an anger. Adolescence is a traumatic time for every child and parent, and a physical disability can add to this. Questions start to be asked which may not have answers, and confidence with the opposite sex or with peer groups may be affected by the person's disability.

These factors are true of any disability, not only of cerebral palsy, but they highlight the problems of growing up with a disability. The disability itself may not develop but the manifestations of it tend to increase as the child grows up. It is possible that during this time, as the young person is growing, they find it increasingly difficult to use their limbs in the way that they did when they were smaller. This can extend the limitations of their movements: fashionable clothes may be more difficult to manage due to small buttons, etc.

As we grow up our priorities in life begin to change. Everyone goes through this transition period, some of us later than others! The adult with cerebral palsy is no different. If we think about the transition from full-time education to a working life, then we can all remember how different the world seemed when you were actually in it. Life began to change, we have to take up responsibility. We also have to take into consideration the possibility of unemployment, accommodation, finances. Whilst we all face these problems, they are even more difficult if a physical disability is added on.

Griffiths and Clegg (1988) identify five areas where consideration should be given for both disabled and able-bodied adolescents:

- self-determination and identity
- independence
- respect and the need to be valued for oneself
- work and appropriate outlets for self-expression
- satisfactory relationships with peers

When we are identifying symptoms and their manifestations the above points must be taken into consideration. They need to provide the basis for beginning to understand how neurological problems show themselves in individuals.

SIGNS AND SYMPTOMS

Cerebral palsy is a complex condition, however, without trying to simplify it in any way, groups of symptoms can be arrived at by looking at the initial diagnosis.

The following outlines the possible symptoms of neurological damage in five main types of cerebral palsy: spastic diplegia, spastic hemiplegia, spastic quadriplegia, athetosis and ataxia. These are by no means simplistic lists; there can be any number of manifestations of symptoms, each one very important to the individual concerned and therefore very important to the conductor working with the individual.

Spastic diplegia

Although there is minimal damage to the **upper arm function**, fine motor functions can often be seen to be clumsy. This can cause specific problems with fashionable clothing, independence in daily living activities and can cause fear and concern with handling a baby.

The greatest problems in motor function are evident in the **lower limbs**. As the person grows in height and weight, the effect of these can increase. Spasticity present in the lower limbs has an effect on the hips, knees and feet.

Hips

The classical clinical picture is of hip-flexion spasm, internal rotation, adduction spasm and contractures. Contractures tend to develop over time, due to lack of mobility, and therefore it is more common to see hip contractures in adults than in children.

Mobility should not be confused with walking. The majority of diplegic adults will be able to walk either with or without an aid. Their gait and posture in walking is of great importance in preventing or causing deformities, contractures and, in some cases, pain.

The upper trunk often leans forward due to lack of extension in the hips, and this can cause further problems in later life, such as back problems due to the strain placed on the lower back to maintain balance. In many cases, as children, there will have been surgical intervention to correct the hips, but this may or may not have relieved the problem.

In adults, surgery may be carried out to relieve pain from deformities. In the absence of surgical procedures, it is possible that the person will cross their legs when stepping, due to the adductor spasm in the hip. If surgical procedures overcompensate for this, then it is possible that they will have a wide gait when walking.

Knees
The knees are often pressed together due to rotation of the hips. They are often held slightly flexed in all positions. This position of the knees can, over a prolonged period, cause pain and deformity in the knee joints. Weight bearing over a flexed joint causes an increase in the strain on the joint and this can cause pain and restrict mobility.

Feet and ankles
Equinus of ankles is seen, usually one side is more affected than the other. Pes valgus and plantar flexed talus are also often present. Deformities are likely, and this can make it very difficult for the person to find shoes which fit. Young adolescents naturally wish to wear fashionable shoes, but in the long term this can increase deformities and any deformity has the potential to cause pain. It is very important that the conductor remains aware of this when working with the adult.

Vision
This type of cerebral palsy carries the largest occurrence of squints. Again, these can be surgically corrected but are often still evident in adulthood.

Perception
There is frequently some form of perceptual disturbance which, if not identified, will have an impact on the ability to learn. If the disturbance is sensory, then it can affect their body image and the fine control over their movements.

Spacial awareness
This is often affected and will disturb the ability to identify objects in space. It can also lead to a lack of fine co-ordination.

Emotional factors
People with spastic diplegia often experience fear and tension. This will not only affect their ability to learn but also their self-confidence, particularly when faced with a new situation. This can be a great social barrier in adulthood.

Spastic hemiplegia

This is the most common form of cerebral palsy. The level of paresis is not the same in all muscles. Generally, there is flexion in upper limbs and extension in lower, the lower limbs being less affected than the upper. The majority of children will learn to walk but this may be delayed. The level of mobility will depend on associative disorders and not purely on motor function.

Upper limbs

There is evidence of the Wernicke Mann position – shoulder towards trunk, elbow flexed, lower arm inwardly rotated, wrist bent, thumb in palm. The degree of damage will vary greatly but it is common that the adult will have limited spontaneous movement in the upper limb on the affected side. Over the years they will have learnt how to compensate by performing activities with one hand.

It is often the case that as life goes on this becomes more and more limiting and the adult tends to want to try and perform some function with the upper limb. After years of lack of use, it is likely that the arm will be less developed than the other one, causing physiological differences in the two arms. There is often a shortening of the limb that makes lateral co-ordination very difficult.

Contractures in the shoulder, elbow, wrists and fingers are very common. Some children may have had surgery to reduce the effect of contractures, more common with the fingers. In adulthood it is quite common to see over-extension of the fingers as a result of corrective surgery. This causes increased difficulty for the person when using their fingers in everyday activities.

There is often a lack of sensation in the affected upper limb, which causes problems with overall body image and can result in a denial of the limb. As with other contractures and deformities, the person may experience some pain. This may be dulled due to lack of sensation, but it is also possible that sensation is heightened.

Lower limbs

As with diplegia, there may be equinus of foot and ankle, and circumduction of the affected leg is also very common. Again there is the risk of deformities in the ankle and foot.

Cognition

Hemiplegics often have low cognitive abilities that affect learning and can cause a severe learning difficulty. This may be more serious than the motor dysfunction.

Behaviour

Behavioural problems are often displayed. These are due to neurological damage and not the personality of the child or adult. Again, these can inhibit learning and the development of skills.

Other

Epilepsy, particularly late-onset, can also occur. In addition, it is possible that there will be some form of aphasia which can affect communication abilities. Lateralization problems are very common, but if they have been helped in childhood then these can usually be overcome by adulthood.

Spastic quadriplegia

As the name suggests it is manifested in all four limbs. Again, the degree of this will vary between individuals. The main characteristics are as follows:

Upper limbs

Limbs are usually in a flexed position, wrists cocked, fingers in a fist, thumb in palm. This severely limits any hand function. The adult is likely to have learnt some hand function but this can still be severely limited, causing difficulties in everyday living skills and restricting independence.

Lower limbs

Limbs are usually flexed, hips adducted, often causing legs to cross. There is likely to be severe atrophy from lack of use, particularly with lower limbs. Deformities of feet are common as they have not developed due to lack of weight bearing. Dislocation of hips is often a common feature in childhood, but the possibility of this lessens in adulthood. Contractures of hips, knees and ankles are very common. The degree of these will depend on the level of active movement and the extent of developmental therapy during childhood.

Other

Dribbling is very frequent and this can be quite excessive and distressing by adulthood. There are surgical procedures to assist with this. There may be problems with tongue control, swallowing and chewing. In extreme cases the individual would need to have a special diet or mashed food.

Lack of facial expression is an underrated symptom. Since it does not affect our ability to perform physical functions, we tend to see it as not significant. On the contrary a lack of facial expression causes severe emotional and social problems. The individual concerned finds it very difficult to form relationships with others as the wrong signals would be given. The effects of this are perhaps greater in adulthood than in childhood; the same is true of dribbling, swallowing and chewing. It is also possible that there will be some form of speech problem that may affect communication.

Epilepsy often occurs in quadriplegia. Although this can be successfully controlled with drugs, the onset of puberty and adolescence can often change the balance and a review of drugs is required. This can take some time to restabilize. Again this has a huge impact on the individual and the family with regard to emotional, social and medical factors.

Quadriplegics often display a lack of motivation and can be very withdrawn. This is not due to the personality of the person or the fact that they are disabled, but is a direct result of neurological damage. It is very common to find these symptoms in adulthood as they have frequently not been a priority in childhood. When we are in a structured learning environment we are more likely to be motivated than when we have to self-motivate. Adulthood tends to bring more situations where a person has to find activities for themselves, motivate themselves. This can be very difficult for quadriplegics and leads to a reduction in activity. They are quite likely to have cognitive problems as well as a lack of spacial awareness.

There are four main positions identified in spastic quadriplegia:

- extensive position – all four limbs are stretched
- flexive position – all four limbs are flexed
- frog position – lower limbs come away from hips
- asymmetric position – one leg rotates inwardly and the other outwards.

The above are clinical pictures and thus often present themselves in mixed forms. Deformities of the spine can result in a lack of appropriate movement and if the person remains in one position for too long. Deformities of the hip are very common in adulthood, sometimes to the extent that the person is unable to remain in a sitting position without being strapped in.

Athetosis

This usually involves all four limbs. It can also be accompanied by involuntary facial gestures. There is a constant change in tone and this results in involuntary movements. These movements are arrhythmic and only stop during sleep.

Athetosis can take many forms and the form in childhood may change during adulthood. As the child tries to stop the involuntary movements their clinical picture can move to one of total rigidity and contractures. An adult with athetosis may not be apparent on first sight, they may have the clinical picture of spastic quadriplegia. On the other hand, a large number will retain the snake-like writhing movements. The following are some of the types of athetosis. They cannot be separated from each other as there are a number of common features.

Tension athetosis
The involuntary movements lead to spasm and a total rigid state can be observed.

Contractive athetosis
This is also characterized by rigidity of the limbs, either in a flexed or extended position. If flexed it is usually very difficult to try and extend them. If they manage to loosen the contracture, chorea athetosis is often seen. This involves a sudden, violent movement of the limb.

Torsion athetosis
The head and neck are twisted to one side and this causes the whole body to twist. This movement is sudden and may be limited to a dystonic movement of the head.

Ballism
Either the upper or lower limbs are affected. Ballism is very rare. Involun-

tary movements increase with a willed, conscious action. They can also be increased by excitement, insecurity or mental concentration. Fluctuating tone sometimes occurs with fluctuating moods.

Other

Other symptoms include problems with swallowing, speech, breathing and chewing. Again all these are very important for social and emotional well-being. There may be evidence of lateral confusion but this is usually overcome by adulthood. Hearing loss caused by kernicterus is common and this cannot be assisted with hearing appliances.

Ataxia

This occurs as the result of damage to the cerebellum. The cerebellum controls our movements in space and time and thus plays a large role in the co-ordination of our movements and our balance. These are two of the main areas that are problematic for the ataxic person. Ataxia can be present in the limbs, trunk or both.

Balance

Due to problems maintaining balance, the ataxic person has a very characteristic gait. Legs are wide apart ensuring a large base for stability, knees are usually extended, in some cases hyper-extended, and arms tend to produce balance-saving reactions. When stepping, feet tend to slap the floor and knees remain stretched. Most will learn to walk but this can be unstable.

Charcot's triad

This is very common with ataxia, and includes staccato speech, intentional tremor and nystagmus.

Other

Ataxia sufferers are often unable to produce movements in rapid succession. Cognitive abilities are frequently affected and the ataxic person tends to have an intellectual level considerably lower than their chronological age. It is quite common that associated dysfunctions other than motor are more disabling than the motor functions for these people.

From the above, we can see that cerebral palsy is a blanket term, that covers almost every possibility for neurological disorder. The adult with cerebral palsy may have the same symptoms as someone who has an acquired disorder, such as multiple sclerosis or a stroke, however the implications will be very different.

During one of our group sessions there was a discussion between two young adults, one who had cerebral palsy and one who had suffered a head injury. The conversation was based around their individual plight. The young man with cerebral palsy said that the other man was more fortunate than him because he had at least had the experience of movement. The other's reply was that this was not true at all; it was better not to have had something than to have it taken away from you!

FROM ADOLESENCE TO ADULTHOOD

It is impossible for the conductor, therapist, doctor or family to make assumptions about the effect of neurological damage on a person. The developmental therapy with a cerebral palsied person tends to finish once schooling is over. This is one of the most vulnerable times in their life. As needs change, priorities change, and as these change the need for intervention changes. We are all continually learning and progressing throughout our lives; our education does not finish with schooling, but rather begins.

The same is true for the cerebral palsied person. Whilst we tend to assume that the person has begun to learn how to cope with the symptoms of their condition, we must also remember that the effects of these will grow with the person into adulthood. Although in childhood it was acceptable for someone to help you to the toilet or bath you, this becomes less so in adulthood. As a child you only went out when accompanied by someone else, but in adulthood this is inconvenient and signifies a loss of independence.

Using a wheelchair may be an enormous step towards independence, but if a person is unable to transfer, then they will be restricted in pubs, night-clubs and possibly in work. Transferring may not have been a priority during childhood but can become one during adulthood.

For many children and their families, walking tends to be a priority. In adulthood, activities such as daily living skills, communication and transferring usually take priority over walking. The conductor must ensure that they are meeting the immediate goals of the person they are working with.

THE CONSULTATION

The conductor may be meeting the person for the first time or the person may have participated in conductive education during their childhood. As with all intervention the earlier it starts the better, but adults with cerebral palsy are not excluded from this system of education.

The consultation will be very important in establishing the priorities of the individual and allowing the conductor to observe any methods the person uses for overcoming daily problems. The conductor must be aware that the adult has had a lifetime of experience of how to deal with the problems and, it is thus very important that the conductor finds a base from which to work. The person is also likely to be seeking assistance in specific areas and these must be discussed in depth.

APPLICATION FORM INFORMATION

Before attending the consultation the person will have completed a basic application form described in Chapter 1. In addition to this, further questions will have been added relevant to adults with cerebral palsy. It is impossible to cover all possible areas of neurological damage, but the questions will act as indicators for the conductor, thus allowing them to prepare in advance.

- the exact diagnosis and age at diagnosis
- presence of tremor, stiffness, involuntary movements
- contractures, noting which joints are affected
- potted medical history of operations and dates
- main method of communicating
- outline of present abilities in specified everyday activities, e.g. dressing, washing, getting in and out of bed, etc.
- educational background, if relevant
- continence problems, if any
- use of aids, appliances, etc.; type and frequency of use
- presence of epilepsy
- vision, hearing difficulties.

ADDITIONAL INFORMATION

Now the conductor will have a clearer picture of the problems faced by the individual and it allows them to prepare a relevant format for the consultation. The person will be asked to bring any aids with them they use regularly, such as communications or walking aids, thus enabling them to function at an appropriate level and also to communicate with the conductor.

Medical reports are essential, particularly if there is evidence of deformities or orthopaedic problems. It may be necessary for the conductor to make contact with the relevant specialist before embarking on a programme, and this will be discussed during the consultation. If the person is still receiving some form of therapy, it is important for the conductor to find out what help is being given and obtain permission from the individual to contact the therapist in order to ensure continuity of provision.

GOALS AND PROVISION

The conductor needs to establish the priorities of the individual and then to assess ways in which conductive education may be able to help with these. In order to do this, a detailed discussion will be led by the conductor regarding the difficulties the person faces and the specific areas they would like help with. Some examples would be to increase overall movement, improve walking technique, help with speech and help with voluntary control of movements.

The adult with cerebral palsy is rarely unrealistic about their goals, if anything they underrate their own potential. If, however, a person **is** setting unrealistic goals for themselves, then the conductor must discuss this with them and inform them that these goals may not be achievable and that smaller, shorter term goals may be more appropriate.

It is impossible to see into the future and to predict someone's potential – we are not even able to do this for ourselves. The conductor must encourage each individual to look at the next step and to set shorter term goals that can lead towards a long-term aim. There are no guarantees, no assurances, and the individual must realise this. However, this, does not preclude the person from being given every available opportunity to realize their own potential.

ASSESSMENT OF MOTOR ABILITIES

The conductor will have been observing the spontaneous movements of the person from the first introduction. A guide to motor abilities and communication abilities will have already been established during the initial discussion, and from this information the conductor will decide which elements of movement they need to see in greater detail.

The main areas the conductor will be observing at this stage are gross movements of legs and arms, fine hand co-ordination, range of movement in joints both passively and actively, awareness of body parts, ability to fix involuntary movements and how this is achieved, and signs of neglect on the affected side if hemiplegic. Overall co-ordination will play a role in the practical assessment.

Basic movements

To evaluate these elements, the conductor will ask the person to perform a few basic movements in a lying position and then, if appropriate, whilst sitting and standing.

The precise nature of these movements will depend on the basic level of the individual, but will include general changing of position, active movement of legs by bending and lifting, the same of arms, moving across from one chair to another, lying down, sitting up, clasping hands, pronation and supination of palms. If the person is able to perform these forms of movement, then the conductor may ask them to stand up, balance on one leg with or without support, crouch down, and so on.

The main role of the conductor during the consultation is to allow the person to display the abilities they still have and they will do this by gradually increasing the difficulty of the task until they find the appropriate level. This will give a guide to the baseline level of that person.

Due to the wide range of problems associated with this diagnosis, it is impossible to give a standard assessment for motor ability, i.e. if the person is finding the tasks very easy then the conductor misses out a few stages; if they have very limited movement then the conductor helps them to perform some basic movements.

During these movements the conductor will also have been able to assess if there are problems with lateralization, body image and comprehension of language. Any joints that appear to have contractures need to be examined further, and the conductor will try and passively move the joint to its full extent. Whilst doing this, the conductor needs to be very observant to ensure that this is not causing pain.

Throughout the movement assessment it is important that the person feels secure. A person with severe athetosis may feel more secure on a mat on the floor than on a plinth, or may need two plinths pushed together. Others may feel very disorientated when lying supine and may need to have someone sitting next to them for security. If the person is unable to lie down securely, the conductor must observe movements in another position. Any deformities of the spine may make it very uncomfortable for the person to lie or sit in certain positions, and the conductor should ask about these and find the most appropriate position for the person.

Other concerns

As mentioned previously the conductor is not only concerned with physical abilities but also cognitive, emotional, social and communication skills. Much of this will be evident as the consultation proceeds. The conductor may request specific activities relating to cognitive or perceptive skills if they feel that this is necessary. There are a number of standard tests available in these areas and the conductor may use one which they are familiar with.

The conductor may also need to ask specifically about continence problems, visual problems, hearing problems, lack of feeling, pain, and so on. Although there will have been an indication of these on the application form it is important that the conductor allows the person an opportunity to discuss the nature and extent of the problems they face. This will give a greater indication of the priority areas for the person.

The consultation will end with the conductor summarizing the problems they have discussed and outlining the type of assistance, if any, that can be given. This will be followed by a discussion on the placement required to meet these needs and the practical arrangements if that person were to attend sessions. A written account of this consultation will also be sent to the person and this gives them time to consider the recommendations and decide if they wish to take up placement.

The consultation, although a very important starting point, is only the beginning of the observation of the person, only the beginning of the process. The conductor needs to work with the person for some time before they are in a position to give concrete information about their skills. The consultation can be a stressful situation, which means that the person will not be able to perform all the movements they are capable of. The conductor must ensure that the person realizes that this is understood and that there will be a continual review of progress and aims once they begin the programme.

The consultation may have been attended by a carer or a member of the family. It is important that they also play a role but that the central role focuses around the prospective participant. In some cases it may be suggested that the carer or family member attends the session with the participant to assist with the continuity in the home situation. This will depend on the individual and needs to be discussed with all parties concerned. In many cases they find this to be a more helpful way of working.

PLANNING THE CONDUCTIVE PROGRAMME

As with all other programme planning, there are two levels – **general** and **individual**. The person concerned may be working as part of a group or may be attending individual sessions with or without a carer. The aims for the person will be the same whether they are in a group or attending individually. The aims will have been set in the discussion during the consultation.

Groups do not run according to diagnosis alone, but rather the effect of the symptoms. As mentioned at the beginning of this chapter, the neurological damage caused by cerebral palsy may be similar to the neurological damage caused by a stroke, head injury or multiple sclerosis. The programme for these groups may also benefit the participant with cerebral palsy. As with head injuries, it is important to consider carefully the implications when placing a person with cerebral palsy in a group where the other members have a progressive condition. The needs of rehabilitation may differ considerably between the groups and this must be discussed with the individuals concerned.

The details of programme planning for these diverse groups are already discussed in other chapters. Previous chapters, in particular those concerning stroke, head injury and multiple sclerosis, in addition to the basic programme outlined in Chapter 12, will give an insight into the relevant programme for people with cerebral palsy.

The baseline level of the individual must be used not only as the starting point but as an indication of the way forward.

FACILITATION

There is no facilitation specified for a diagnostic group, however there are many guidelines the conductor should use when facilitating a participant.

It is likely that the adult with cerebral palsy will be using a number of aids to assist with their mobility. It is not the aim of conductive education to remove these as this would in fact de-skill the person and not add to their present skill level.

ORTHOFUNCTION

Griffiths (1988) described conductive education as helping a person to overcome dysfunction and achieve orthofunction, which means functioning in a normal society without the use of aids or wheelchairs. This is not a true representation of conductive education. It would be impossible to set out with this aim as the large majority of people would never achieve it. In addition, conductive education is based on setting realistic goals, not idealistic goals.

Orthofunction as a concept is widely used in literature about conductive education and yet it is widely misunderstood. Orthofunction means living with maximum independence and using full potential to achieve this. This will differ daily and will depend on the activity at hand: if the aim is to go shopping, then it may be appropriate for the person to use a wheelchair; if the aim is to weight bear through the legs, then it would not be appropriate; if the aim is to improve articulation, a communication aid would not be appropriate; if the aim is to increase social skills, then a communication aid may be relevant and help to achieve the aim.

Orthofunction cannot be described as a simple statement, it is a process where the person is performing an activity with maximum independence and minimum assistance. Not only will this change according to the aim, but also according to the time of day.

AIMS OF FACILITATION

Facilitation is used to enable a person to actively perform a task or activity, and it is based on the ability of the individual together with the next stage of learning. It will depend on the task at hand and the individual aim of the person.

Facilitation can take many forms; physical assistance is always minimal and the last form of facilitation used. It is likely that the person with cerebral palsy may need physical assistance to help secure other limbs whilst they are working with one.

As has been said throughout the book, the test of a facilitation is whether it can be removed. This does not mean that it will be removed immediately but that it promotes learning. If there is no learning then the facilitation remains.

AIDS AND APPLIANCES

The same is true of aids and appliances: they should promote learning. There are two main functions of any aid: to assist movement and to replace movement.

It is very important that movements are not replaced too early and that they are only **assisted**. This becomes particularly true when we see young adolescents who have used a wheelchair from an early age and wish to improve their mobility, to learn how to stand, transfer and take a few steps, and this will happen due to a change in priorities. It is therefore essential that all basic movements are performed from time to time and all possibilities are kept open for that person. This has to be done without creating false hopes. Once movements are replaced then the chance of being able to use them in the future will be reduced.

On the other hand, this does not mean that aids should not be used. They must be used to promote independence and activity. It is more important for someone to gain independence than to be stuck at home unable to move around.

The same is true of **how** the person moves. In all cases movement is preferable to no movement. Once a person is active then movements can be guided and corrected, none of us wait until we can perfect a skill before trying it. The process of learning begins with action and finishes with skill.

The introduction of aids is a sensitive issue, and should not be seen as giving up but rather as enhancing learning. This can only be done, however, if aids are seen as assisting and not replacing movements and independence. Facilitation for the person with cerebral palsy will hinge on the appropriate use of aids as well as promoting active management of skill.

The reader should refer to Chapter 6 for more detailed discussion on the use of aids and equipment. Alongside this, other forms of facilitation as discussed in Chapter 1 should be employed by the conductor to promote learning and thereby increase the level of skill of the participant.

SUMMARY

This chapter has outlined the manifestations of cerebral palsy in adulthood. As priorities change so must the overall aims. It is, however, very important to maintain as wide a range of movements as possible, as this will give a base to allow a change in goals as needs change. The person should not be disadvantaged by using aids to replace movement but given maximum advantages by using aids and facilitation to assist movement.

The effect of disability on adults is very different to its effect on children and this must be taken into consideration by the conductor. The individual must have control over their own learning process. The conductor will ensure this by regularly reviewing progress and discussing difficulties with the individual concerned.

Cerebral palsy not only affects motor abilities, but associated dysfunctions can cause greater problems than the motor dysfunction and this must be taken into consideration. The programme needs to include elements for all skills and help to maintain the level of skill that the person already has. Realistic goals should be set to encourage success and to lead to greater self-confidence and motivation.

Conductive education aims to teach the adult with cerebral palsy how to use the skills they have in the most effective way, and how to remain active to reduce the possibility of deformities. Learning takes place in small stages, but each stage will be of importance to the individual and this must not be underestimated.

The programme for the adult with cerebral palsy will be varied according to the specific problems the individual faces and not necessarily in line with a particular diagnosis. For further information on basic programmes, the reader should refer to the programmes for other diagnoses and find the one most suitable for the group or person they are working with.

Adults with cerebral palsy can benefit from conductive education as well as children. The system needs to be applied to the basic needs of the person and this will take into consideration age, abilities and lifestyle.

Basic task series 12

This chapter aims to provide the basic elements for various task series according to the main diagnoses discussed in this section. Individual tasks are not included as these will depend on the group but the overall structure of the task series can be used as a guide for the conductor.

The task series included are:

- Parkinson's disease
- multiple sclerosis
- head injury
- stroke
- cerebral palsy.

These task series are a guide and can be varied if necessary. They include only the motor elements of the tasks and should be used in conjunction with the information provided throughout this book. The framework should be completed in detail for each group before group sessions begin.

PARKINSON'S DISEASE

Below are the basic tasks in the task series for Parkinson's disease groups, based on a 90 minute session.

LYING TASK SERIES

This task series usually lasts approximately 30 minutes.

1. Sitting up, lying down.
2. Movement to each side.
3. Bending of legs, alternate and simultaneous.
4. Movements of arms, including fine movements.
5. Complex movements of arms and legs, unilaterally, bilaterally.

6. Sitting up in varying directions.
7. Movements of arms and legs in stretched position, in varying directions.
8. Moving from sitting to standing.
9. Kneeling, crouching down.
10. Movements of feet and toes.

TABLE TASK SERIES

These tasks are carried out sitting at a table, and last approximately 20 minutes.

1. Standing up, sitting down.
2. Gross movements of upper limbs.
3. Finer movements of upper limbs.
4. Complex movements, including gross and fine movements.
5. Movements involving changing rhythm, increasing and decreasing.
6. Movements involving supination and pronation of wrists.
7. Changing weight-bearing position in standing.

PREPARATION FOR WRITING

This task usually lasts 10 minutes, followed by a practical writing activity of 5 minutes.

1. Movements of hands, alternate and simultaneous.
2. Movements of fingers in varying directions, performed with one hand and both hands, each finger in turn.
3. Pronation and supination of wrists.
4. Movements to teach sliding of wrists along paper.
5. Work with pencils, grip, fine movements.
6. Complex movements with one and both hands.
7. Writing practice (patterns, letter formation, dictation or copying).

FACIAL TASKS

These last approximately 5 minutes. The participants should be sitting with a mirror in front of them.

1. Movements of individual parts of face.
2. Combination of movements with breathing tasks.
3. Practice of expression.
4. Articulation practice, with rhythm.

POSTURAL TASKS AND PREPARATION FOR WALKING

These take approximately 10 minutes, and should be performed sitting on a chair.

1. Moving from sitting to standing position.
2. Movements of head and shoulders, whilst in standing and sitting.
3. Changing balance point whilst standing.
4. Movements of legs in all directions, whilst sitting.
5. Combination of movements of arms and legs.
6. Tasks to assist size of step, in all directions.
7. Lifting of knees.
8. Movements of ankles and toes.
9. Tasks involving change of rhythm.

WALKING TASKS

This series takes approximately 10 minutes, in a standing position.

1. Stepping in all directions.
2. Movement of arms whilst stepping.
3. Tasks to improve ability to balance.
4. Tasks to improve weight bearing from one foot to the other.
5. Tasks to encourage arm swing whilst walking.
6. Continuous walking, changing direction, stepping backwards.
7. Tasks which help to cope with obstacles whilst maintaining walking rhythm.

The sessions always end with breathing tasks, which help to 'warm down'. All the other elements of conductive programmes should be built in throughout.

MULTIPLE SCLEROSIS

This task series is based on a 90 minute group session. The following is a basic framework the conductor will need to build up to suit the needs of the group in question. For an individual session, the conductor would use this basic task series to cover the specific needs of the person concerned.

Much of the tasks series will be executed in a lying position. This gives the person security within which to correct movements, as well as providing a good position for learning to relax and reduce spasticity. It enables the person to correct their position without having to work against gravity and has a direct effect on their upright position.

LYING TASK SERIES

This series lasts for approximately 50 minutes.

1. Tasks to bend and stretch legs, alternately and simultaneously.
2. Tasks to loosen hips, e.g. relaxing knee/s to the sides.
3. Rolling to both sides and balancing in this position.
4. Lifting legs in all directions whilst supine and lying on each side.
5. Breathing tasks to help increase/maintain lung capacity and help with continence.
6. Tasks in prone position, including movement of arms and legs.
7. Kneeling position for balance. Moving limbs in this position.
8. Aiming movements of hands and fingers.
9. Moving from lying position to sitting with legs stretched out in front.
10. Moving from sitting to standing, with or without support.

STANDING TASKS

These tasks are usually performed for about 5 minutes from a chair facing the plinth for added security.

1. Moving from sitting to standing with minimum support.
2. Tasks to increase flexibility of hips and ankles in a standing position. The person uses support if required.
3. Sitting down on chairs of varying heights according to individual ability.

HAND TASKS

These tasks take approximately 15 minutes and can be done sitting on the edge of the plinth or on a chair, depending on the level of abilities of the group. All participants should be in the same position for these, i.e. on plinth or chair. Some of these tasks may be completed with eyes closed.

1. Tasks including movement of wrists – pronation, supination, flexion, extension, rotation.
2. Tasks to include transference of weight and sitting balance, e.g. leaning forward and sitting up using upper trunk.
3. Tasks involving precision of fine movements, e.g. finger to nose, fist to forehead. All these are done with each finger in turn.
4. Tasks with a small baton/stick – lifting up, holding with index finger and thumb and changing fingers, leaning forward and placing on the floor.
5. Tasks involving gross and fine movements, e.g. lifting arm and circling one finger at a time.

These tasks can be repeated in different ways, and it is important that each element in many variations is included. The emphasis of each element will depend on the group, but each of the above elements must be present.

EYE TASKS

These should be included with all groups and take approximately 5 minutes.

1. Focus on a near point and then move focus to a more distant point.
2. Focus on an object which is then moved by the conductor and the eyes follow it.
3. Focusing and tracking the index finger.

PREPARATION FOR WALKING

This is an extension of the task series previously carried out in a lying and sitting position. This series is carried out mainly in a sitting position and takes about 10 minutes.

1. Lifting knees and extending knees.
2. Tasks to teach appropriate stepping position forwards and to the side.
3. Tasks to improve movement of ankles in all directions.
4. Tasks to ensure transference of weight, e.g. putting right heel on left knee, etc.
5. Practise moving from sitting into standing position.
6. Transference of weight in a standing position.

WALKING TASKS

These tasks take about 5 minutes and will depend on the individual abilities of each person. They may be carried out with support or alone. The eyes may be closed in some cases, but only if balance has been achieved with eyes open. The aim of the walking programme is two-fold:

- to improve the present way of moving around
- to learn how to move around with decreased support, thus enabling the individual to practise the next stage of walking with support.

HEAD INJURY

This task series is based on a 90 minute group session. The following is a framework within which the conductor will work to ensure a programme suitable for each individual in the group. Much of this task series would be executed in a lying position as this ensures a secure position for the individual and also allows for reduction in spasticity.

LYING TASK SERIES

These tasks last for approximately 60 minutes.

1. Transferring across from wheelchair, if appropriate.
2. Tasks to learn how to bend and stretch limbs simultaneously and individually.
3. Tasks to teach basic change of position, e.g. rolling to one side, moving from prone to supine, sitting up, etc.
4. Tasks to increase range of movement in all four limbs, e.g. taking legs apart, arms to the sides, arms above head, etc.
5. Tasks to increase symmetry of body position and movements, e.g. tasks with clasped hands, holding a baton, etc.
6. Breathing tasks can include elements of speech if required.
7. Tasks in a prone position with arms and legs (depending on the abilities of group, use of catheter, etc.).

Tasks should be varied to enhance learning. The basic movements above can be performed in many ways and in different combinations.

TRANSFERRING OR STANDING TASKS

These tasks should last approximately 10 minutes.

1. Tasks to teach active transference from different and to different heights.
2. Tasks to improve standing balance.
3. Tasks to teach standing up from chairs of varying height.

At the end of these tasks time can be given, if required, for putting on shoes, tying laces, etc., all of which assist sitting balance.

HAND TASKS

Hand tasks should be carried out for approximately 10 minutes.

1. Tasks to assist sitting balance.
2. Tasks to increase range of movement with upper body.
3. Tasks to increase finer movements of wrists, hands and fingers.
4. Practical tasks requiring cognitive and physical skills.
5. Breathing tasks, accompanied with arm movements.

INDIVIDUAL TASKS

These tasks last approximately 10 minutes and take into consideration any individual aims requiring further input, e.g. walking, speech, language and cognitive, perceptual or visual activities. These tasks will be determined by the composition of the group, and it may be more appropriate to perform these activities with the whole group.

STROKE

This task series is based on a 90 minute group programme excluding the time taken to walk into the room. If work is with an individual, then the appropriate tasks should be taken from this base, working for no longer than 60 minutes.

WALKING INTO ROOM

This series lasts approximately 5 minutes. Each individual should walk into the room (if they are ambulant), with support if needed. The aim of this is to establish symmetry and to teach them to bear weight on the affected limb. Their walking should be taken on to the next stage at this point: if they walk with a stick then they should walk with the conductor supporting if necessary.

It is very important that all tasks are carried out with both sides of the body. The participant should be encouraged to use the non-affected side to provide the picture of the movement. They must be encouraged to perform tasks accurately and slowly with the non-affected side.

LYING TASK SERIES

These tasks take approximately 45 minutes, but can be reduced depending on the severity of the group members.

1. Tasks to teach reduction of spasticity in upper limb. This may include use of gravity.
2. Tasks including flexion and extension of lower limbs.
3. Tasks to increase range of movement of upper limbs, including tasks with clasped hands.
4. Tasks to teach simultaneous movement of upper and lower limbs.
5. Tasks to improve breathing technique and enhance reduction of spasticity.
6. Tasks transferring the body in all positions to both the affected and non-affected side.
7. Tasks to increase the range of adduction and abduction of limbs on affected side.
8. Hand tasks in all positions, possibly using a baton, clasped hands or hands alone.

All the above tasks promote symmetry and improve overall body awareness. Visual feedback on the affected side is very important for these groups, particularly if there is sensory loss or loss of field of vision.

HAND TASKS

Again, these tasks will depend on the severity of the participants and the necessity to perform hand tasks in a lying position. The series should take about 15 minutes.

Participants should be sitting at a table and be able to place elbows on the table and feet flat on the floor.

1. Tasks to increase symmetry of upper limbs.
2. Tasks to teach pronation and supination of wrist.
3. Tasks to teach grasp and release.
4. Tasks to teach differentiated finger movements.

FACIAL TASKS

These tasks take approximately 5 minutes and can be carried out sitting at a table with a mirror.

1. Breathing tasks of varying kinds including formation of vowel sounds.
2. Movements of eye, cheek and mouth on affected side.
3. Tasks to involve movement of the tongue in all directions.

SITTING TASKS INCLUDING PREPARATION FOR WALKING

This series of tasks takes approximately 15 minutes.

1. Tasks to include standing up from sitting and vice versa.
2. Tasks to improve balance and weight-bearing in a sitting position.
3. Tasks to include plantar and dorsal flexion of ankle.
4. Tasks to include movement of leg in all directions – lifting, forwards, to the side.
5. Tasks to increase the range of hip movement in all directions.
6. Tasks to improve posture.
7. Tasks using lower limbs separately and simultaneously.
8. Tasks involving upper and lower limbs.

STANDING AND WALKING

These tasks take approximately 10 minutes.

1. Tasks in standing position to teach transference of weight.
2. Tasks to increase balance in a standing position.
3. Tasks to improve symmetry of standing and walking.
4. Walking tasks should be adapted to suit the needs of the individual. If possible tasks should be performed as a group, but individual tasks can be given at this time if necessary.

5. Tasks to include practical aspects of walking, e.g. up and down stairs, swinging arms, around objects, etc.

These tasks are based on a group who have overcome some of their problems and are able to bear weight on their lower limbs. Specific tasks would have to be set at the level of the group and take into consideration other problems that may occur, such as aphasia, loss of visual field, etc.

CEREBRAL PALSY

It is difficult to present a basic task series for the participants as it will be dependent on their previous experience, orthopaedic implications and severity of condition. The following task series should be seen as a baseline that can be added to or taken away from in order to produce a task series beneficial to the group or individual.

The task series is based on a group session of 90 minutes.

LYING TASK SERIES

These tasks can be carried out in approximately 60 minutes.

1. Tasks to teach transferring of body position into lying and when lying.
2. Tasks to teach reduction of spasticity, including breathing tasks.
3. Tasks to increase the range of movement of lower limbs.
4. Tasks to teach a range of movement of upper limbs.
5. Tasks to teach fixing of limbs if athetoid or ataxic.
6. Tasks to teach simultaneous movements of upper and lower limbs.
7. Sitting up in all directions.
8. Rolling to each side.
9. Lifting legs in all directions, or sliding if appropriate.

HAND TASKS

These tasks can be varied if necessary and should take approximately 20 minutes.

1. Tasks involving pronation and supination of wrists.
2. Tasks involving maintenance of sitting balance.
3. Tasks involving symmetry of hand movements, including tasks with clasped hands.
4. Tasks involving grasp and release, if necessary.
5. Tasks involving differentiated finger movements.
6. Gross movements of upper body in all directions.
7. Transferring from sitting position, either to another chair or into a standing position.

SITTING TASKS INCLUDING PREPARATION FOR STANDING AND WALKING.

These tasks, lasting approximately 10 minutes, should only be done if appropriate. If required, tasks can also be taken from the basic task series for head injury or multiple sclerosis.

1. Tasks involving movement of lower limbs in all directions.
2. Tasks including plantar and dorsal flexion of ankles.
3. Tasks including transference of weight in a standing position.
4. Tasks including walking on different surfaces, up and down stairs, etc.

If walking tasks are not appropriate for the individual, then tasks for speech, additional tasks in a sitting position, cognitive tasks, etc. can be built in to complete the programme. It may be that the last part of the session is left for individual tasks if this is more suitable.

SUMMARY

This chapter has outlined some of the basic programmes used for different groups of participants. These can only be used in conjunction with the other chapters in Part 1 and Part 2 of this book.

These task series are not fixed, and they serve to work towards the aims set by the participants and the conductors. It is very important that a task series meets all the aims of the individuals in any one group.

In order to lead a task series, the conductor will have to make use of varying forms of facilitation. This will enable the group to work together as a whole. Each task should be seen as a base that the conductor will build up for some individuals or break down for others. The task, however, remains common to the group.

The rhythm of these task series must be carefully set by the conductor. The conductor must see the rhythm of the whole programme and not just of the individual tasks within the series. The structure of the tasks will be dependent on the appropriate rhythm for the group. It is important that the conductor plans the programme so that the timing of each section of the task series is maintained.

The task series planned for each group must be flexible enough to accommodate any changes that may occur. It may be that the conductor will wish to place an emphasis on one area of motor skill and therefore may spend more time on that part of the task series. It is very important that the conductor does not build a task series that only allows movements of one part of the body or developments in one area only. The task series must be broad enough to cover all aspects of development.

The tasks in this chapter should provide a basis for programme planning. All other elements must be built in by the individual conductor according to their knowledge and experience.

PART THREE

The Personal View

Study of subjects with Parkinson's disease

13

A SUBJECTIVE STUDY

All too often we feel that the subjective view does not offer us scientific evidence of the effectiveness of a service, and yet we must accept that any disability will affect each individual in a different way. Thus, when measuring outcomes, we must first ascertain how the disability affects that individual and then assess any changes.

For those of us in the field of education and rehabilitation the daily activities of the person are uppermost; the effect of disability on the individual can only be truly assessed by the individual themselves, their families and their carers. This voice should not be dismissed as it is the most accurate form of evidence of the benefits of a service provision. Basic economics show that supply equals demand, demand is consumer-led and not led by the supplier. So, in listening to our service users, we must remember that they are the ones who create demand. If a product is not beneficial then demand will fall.

This study was carried out at the National Institute of Conductive Education (formerly the Birmingham Institute for Conductive Education), and followed 13 people with Parkinson's disease over a period of 12 months.

SUBJECTS OF THE STUDY

Subjects for this study were self-selected and each one participated in the programme. Subjects attended between two or three times a week for the period. Each session lasted for 90 minutes.

Table 13.1 Age groups of subjects

Age in years	No. of subjects
40–50	1
51–60	4
61–70	6
71+	2

The initial trial was carried out on the 19 participants in attendance at the time of the study in 1991-1992. Six participants left the institute: one died, three left due to ill-health not related to Parkinson's disease, one due to work commitments and one had a spinal operation.

Of the 13 subjects, three were female and 10 male. The age groups were as outlined in Table 13.1.

Table 13.2 shows the length of time since diagnosis, before attending the Institute.

Table 13.2 Time since diagnosis

Years	No. of subjects
1–5	3
6–10	5
11–15	4
26+	1

Periods of the waking day where the person was 'off' were also monitored, together with freezing when walking. These were taken from the Parkinson's Unified Scale and the scores shown in Table 13.3 and 13.4.

Table 13.3 'Off' periods of waking day and subjects displaying 'freezing'.

'Off' period (%)	No. of subjects
0–6	6
1–25	4
26–50	3

Freezing	No. of subjects
Did not freeze whilst walking	7
Rare freezing	2
Occasional freezing	1
Falling due to freezing	3

These levels were asked for in December 1992, at the end of the study. The subjects reported no difference in their general level of freezing or 'off' periods during the course of the study. They did report that their ability to overcome these two problems had increased and, although the length of time was the same, they were more able to cope.

METHODS OF STUDY

In July 1991 participants were given a short questionnaire relating to their daily activities. This consisted of 13 questions aimed at various sections of everyday life. Scoring was graded between 1 and 7, where 1 was poor and 7 was excellent. The participants were asked to fill in any changes noticed before conductive education and since attendance at the Institute, a period of one year.

This form was filled in by the participants themselves. After discussion with the participants a more detailed questionnaire was produced (Appendix). This contained 11 sections, each one being divided into several parts.

It was felt that the questionnaire covered the main activities of daily living in enough detail to monitor any changes. Other scales, more widely recognized, were also investigated. Hoehn and Yahr scale (1967) was felt to be too vague and therefore of little relevance to this study. The Parkinson's Unified Scale (Fahn and Elton, 1987) covered most of the daily living skills covered in our questionnaire, but there was not enough detailed information in this scale to monitor any significant changes. In addition, aspects such as freezing, 'on' and 'off' periods were not taken into account.

In March 1992, each participant completed the Beck Index (Beck et al., 1964) as a scale for measuring depression. It is often felt that depression in people suffering from Parkinson's disease is of a higher level than for the average population. We found no indication of this with our subjects. It was felt that perhaps this was due to the fact that these people were involved in an active programme and may not have been a true representation of the Parkinson's disease population. For this reason this index was not repeated.

In addition to the questionnaire mentioned above drug levels over the period of the study were also monitored as well as writing samples.

RESULTS

Out of a total of 13 subjects there was an overall increase in performance, as measured by the total score on our revised scale, between December 1991 and December 1992 of 26.34%. Of the 13 subjects, seven improved their overall scores and six did not. We looked at the age of onset and the present age to see if there was any pattern. The highest levels of improvement came from subjects over the age of 70 and under the age of 50, together with those diagnosed less than four years previously and those diagnosed more than 10 years ago.

Out of the seven people who showed improvement there was only one change in level of drugs and that was an increase of 5 mg of procyclidine. Of the six people who regressed, there was one increase of Sinemet plus. It does not appear that changes in drugs had any significant effect on the

Table 13.4 Patterns of performance

Length of diagnosis (years)	No. of subjects	Improved	Regressed
1–4	3	2	1
5–9	5	3	2
10+	5	2	3

conclusions drawn from the study. Eleven of the 13 subjects had maintained their level of drugs over the 12 month period.

Looking at individual sections of the questionnaire, out of the 11 areas identified, improvement was shown in the average score for seven of these. The areas of lying, sitting, bathing and memory showed a decrease in the average scores.

Table 13.5 Percentage differential for each area of questionnaire

Differential (%)	Area of function
– 1.31	Lying
– 7.08	Sitting
+ 1.54	Standing
+ 0.75	Speech
+ 1.62	Reading
– 3.57	Memory
+ 3.16	Writing
– 1.71	Bathing
+ 6.72	Dressing
+ 4.19	Eating
+ 2.28	Self-help

If the percentage differential for all 11 functions is calculated, then a score of + 6.59 is shown.

For the four functions with minus scores we calculated the numbers of subjects scoring above the average difference over the period measured.

Table 13.6 Functions with minus scores

Function	No. of subjects achieving more than average difference over time	%
Lying	9	69.23
Sitting	9	69.23
Memory	11	84.61
Bathing	6	46.15

Thus we identified that the greatest percentage of subjects were in fact above this average. However, those who were below it had fallen greatly. The difference in performance between men and women was also looked at, but it was felt that the results were of no significance from such a small-scale study. The results found did not display any pattern and further subjects would be required to look into this area.

COMMENTS ON FINDINGS OF STUDY

The people who showed improvement tended to show a steady improvement. Those who regressed often showed a sudden deterioration.

One of the greatest problems found was that during the course of conductive education the participants gradually became aware of activities that they were unable to do. In the years previous to the course they had gradually stopped performing certain activities, but the change had been so gradual that they had not noticed the details of it. Their lifestyle had accommodated these changes. There were activities they thought they could perform, but when they tried they found that they were unable to do them. This often resulted in the scores they gave themselves when first completing the questionnaire being higher than their actual scores. This gave rise to a supposed deterioration that had not in fact happened.

Another problem faced was that of self-image and self goals. Throughout the course the person is encouraged to accept the challenge of daily activities. Once they realize that some of the problems can be overcome, they increase their own expectations of self. This meant that over the course of the year the value of 7 on the scale had a different meaning than in the first instance. This was one of the biggest problems we faced and one which makes any subjective study very difficult to quantify.

Unfortunately there was no baseline for results as the participants had already attended sessions for one year prior to the completion of the first questionnaire. The above study, therefore, cannot be seen as an indication of the effectiveness of conductive education, but can give a guide as to the possibilities of teaching someone with a progressive condition to maintain their activity level over a given period of time. A significant point which was highlighted was that the majority of people were able to maintain their condition without requiring an increase in the level of drugs.

In general there was a pattern of some improvement for people who have a progressive condition. There is no way of knowing what would have happened if these people had not attended the sessions, therefore we cannot conclude that conductive education influenced these results. It should be pointed out that none of the subjects was receiving any other form of intervention apart from drugs during the period of the study.

Case studies

14

There follows a selection of case studies of people who have attended the National Institute of Conductive Education. Much of the information has been written by them, but names have been changed to protect the identity of the individuals concerned.

CATHERINE

Catherine, from Cheltenham, was born in 1940 and at the age of 46 began to notice some changes in her ability to use her right hand. One year later she was diagnosed with Parkinson's disease. Over the next few years she was able to remain active and look after her teenage children at home. She found that her movements were beginning to become more difficult and attended for a consultation in June 1992.

AT CONSULTATION

At the time of her consultation the tremor in Catherine's right hand was noticeable and there were few spontaneous movements with this hand. She found it very difficult to flick her thumb and index finger with her right hand. She was still living independently and able to drive. Her overall movements were slow and slightly laboured. When walking, her right arm tended to stay by her side, her left one was swinging in line with her stepping. Her right foot 'stuck' a little to the floor when stepping. She had stiffness and a reduction of movement in her right shoulder and her neck. She lacked some facial expression and her writing, although legible, was slow and the size of the letters slightly reduced.

At the time of her consultation, the main aim was to enable Catherine to maintain her condition by using a minimum level of drugs. At the time she was taking 10 mg of selegiline and 2 mg of benzhexol daily. It was felt that we would be able to teach her to learn how to gain some control over her tremor, increase the spontaneous movements of her right arm, improve her facial expression, assist in maintaining her writing and generally increase the rhythm of her movements.

GROUP WORK FOR CATHERINE

Catherine joined a group that was already established. The others in the group were also displaying minimal symptoms of Parkinson's disease and were following a complex set of tasks with a brisk rhythm. The aim of the whole group was to maintain and slightly increase the rhythm of their movements and increase overall body awareness to improve finer movements.

Catherine became an active member of the group very quickly and was able to follow the programme after the first few sessions. After the first 10 sessions she was beginning to show signs of improvement. Her facial expression was appropriate in both practise and spontaneous situations. Her writing became slightly larger and the pressure used had increased. Her balance was improving and she was more able to bear weight securely on her right foot; this had reduced the 'sticking' when walking. There was an overall increase in the confidence of her movements and she was aware of how she was performing them and the corrections required to maximize her own abilities.

Catherine has continued to attend on a regular basis, and since 1995 this has been reduced from twice a week to once a week. Over this period she has been able to maintain the initial improvements seen, although this requires more concentration.

Catherine still needs to concentrate on performing her movements accurately and needs to maintain the rhythm of her movements. She is still on the same level of drugs and still leads an independent and active life style. Now into her tenth year suffering from Parkinson's disease, she still drives, lives alone and travels, making a 150 mile round trip to attend the institute once a week.

Whilst there is no way of knowing how Catherine's condition would have progressed with only drug therapy, she feels that conductive education has assisted her to maintain her movements and quality of life. She feels that she still needs the regular sessions to help her to correct her movements and is then able to apply this to her other activities during the week.

There has been no dramatic improvement in her condition and abilities, and each day remains a battle to maintain the level of movement skill she has. In spite of having a progressive condition, Catherine is able to complete the majority of activities she wishes to and live a quality life. It is hoped that this will continue.

Figures 14.1, 14.2 and 14.3 show Catherine with a few others in her group

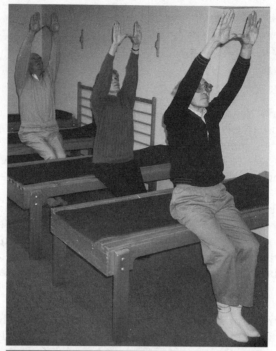

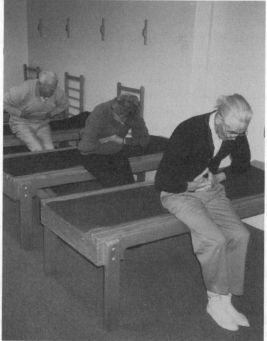

Fig. 14.1–3 (above and opposite) Catherine working with her group

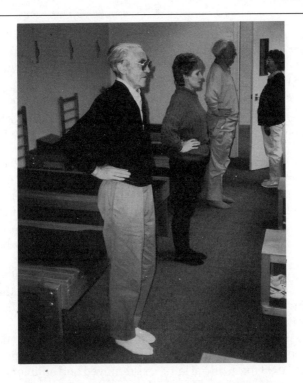

working on positions to help to fix tremor and maximize balance and range of movements.

JAMES

JAMES'S HISTORY

James was born in 1932 and is presently living in Lapworth. In 1969 he had a car accident resulting in a head injury. Following this accident he was left with right hemiparesis and a depressed fracture of the left temporal lobe. There was evidence of clotting inside the lobe and he had an emergency operation to remove this.

James's speech and reading were affected by this accident and, although able to communicate, frequently said the wrong word. There were a number of words he was unable to articulate. On release from hospital there was a question mark about the long-term effect of this accident on his speech. It was felt that although intellectual recovery would be excellent his speech difficulties would inhibit this to some degree. Prior to his accident he was a graduate in languages and spoke many foreign languages.

Following this accident James largely recovered and was able to return to work for a company where he took part in 'un-demanding' work. There were still marked difficulties with his speech and reading, but he overcame these as best he could.

In 1989 James was diagnosed as having Non-Hodgkin's lymphoma. In 1990 he had emergency surgery to remove an 'obstruction' from his spine. In the hours preceding the operation brain damage was reported, and it was felt that he would not be able to walk again. He made a good recovery and within two years he was able to walk a mile or so with the aid of a walker.

In June 1992 James suffered a 'mysterious' car accident. This left him with a complicated fracture of the right hip. He was unconscious for approximately four hours following the crash. His leg was non-weight bearing for three months. At the end of this period he fell, fracturing the hip in another place, and had to undergo another operation. In October 1992 following spontaneous dislocation of the hip, he had a hip replacement.

In January 1993 he was suffering recurrent blackouts, diagnosed as temporal lobe epilepsy. It was felt that a seizure had caused the previous car accident, the cause of the epilepsy being attributed to the car accident 20 years previously.

In February 1993 James was suffering from much pain and reduced movement in his hip caused by an infection which was damaging the bone. In December 1993 the artificial joint was removed and antibiotic applied to the bone. In March 1994 the hip was declared free of infection. He had had no hip for this period and been totally non-weight bearing. In July 1994 a hip replacement was performed, and he received hydrotherapy and physiotherapy for six weeks following surgery.

AT CONSULTATION

In November 1994 James attended for a consultation. At this time he was reliant on a wheelchair but was able to take a few steps with his stick. His walking was asymmetrical, he had spasticity in both his right arm and leg, and the movements of his right leg were reduced with no significant movement of the right ankle.

In addition to physical difficulties, he had lateralization problems and found expressive language difficult. He was unable to name body parts and follow movement instructions. There was some facial paralysis on the right side.

He attended for individual sessions once a week from the time of his consultation. The aim at this time was to try and increase the range of movements on his right side. It was unknown how much his receptive language would improve due to the 25 year time-lag since his original head injury. At the time of the consultation James's main problems were ortho-paedic and not neurological; he was therefore taken on a reviewable basis.

WHAT JAMES SAID ABOUT CONDUCTIVE EDUCATION

Since that time James has continued to attend once weekly on a regular basis. He has worked both individually and as a member of a group. Following one year of provision, James and his wife tried to summarize the changes they had found. The following is an extract from their notes. James spoke into a tape and his wife transcribed this for him.

> I was introduced to conductive education at a college where I had been employed both in an executive and voluntary capacity. I had been given a (second) hip replacement in July 1994 and I knew that in the months ahead my walking would get better. But I was disappointed how slowly this was happening and it was difficult for me to walk for five minutes without getting enormous pain. In the first month of conductive education I found it easier to start and keep going longer. This was partly because I was determined to walk better even though the pain was there. But what I found was a complete interest in my problem. I'd had physiotherapy many times before but what I found now was a real interest in what I was trying to do.
>
> We work as a small group and so there isn't the feeling that you're a complete waste yourself when you see someone having difficulty doing what I can do fairly straight forwardly. The bed used in conductive education is hard and I was afraid that perhaps I would not be able to do this because of the pain. But in the week this became less important. More important was to use the right leg better; trying to get it to move up and down and left to right and also to try to use the left as much as the right. The whole of one's body was being used not just the parts that needed help. Difficult to understand at first but very sensible. The repeating weekly of helping has changed my body. I can do things on my own bed I couldn't have done before and I do things more easily and better. I can stand for half an hour now and not worry too much about the pain. In the garden I walk better. It is early times for me to see the change and perhaps by next year I can say more about it. I want to say that it's made my mind as well as physically much better than it was before.

His wife added:

> We had both become nervous as a result of the disasters of previous years; I know that I was deliberately discouraging him from stretching himself because of my fears of what might happen. We have both recovered a degree of confidence as a result of the conductive education experience and this has been liberating. I endorse everything he says about the improvement in many areas. I noticed in transcribing his tape an improvement in his ability to express himself concisely. He still seems to need a superfluity of words when he's embarking on a topic.

In 1996 the following comments were made by his wife:

> After a year, I see outstanding progress in these areas:
> BALANCE He has greater control of all his movements; getting out of a chair, sitting down and walking. This is a great aid to mobility. I am much less nervous when he is walking.
> BREATHING Last winter he had a chronic cough and was prescribed a course of antibiotics almost at monthly intervals. His posture when sitting is much better and he is always conscious of the need to straighten up. He also practises deep breathing regularly.
> READING For more than 10 years he has read aloud to me daily for up to half an hour. There has been a marked improvement in recent weeks in the speed and fluency of his reading. Somehow he reads more 'naturally'.

James himself summed up his progress to date and his feelings about the sessions he has been attending.

> I am treating myself as a student, learning again a lot of things that I would never have tried to do before. We started in December 1994 and I had the first three weeks with Agi on her own. After that, in January, it was a group. I know that in the first month it was very much better for me than ever I thought and as a result of that I have carried on weekly, continually using my body better and also my intention to do things on other parts of the body is important.
>
> When I went in to have my hip replacement I never thought it would be a long time before I would walk again. To be told by a good consultant that I would not really be able to walk all that much again and to think in terms of the wheelchair surprised me.
>
> To meet people in the conductive education and to suggest that a lot of things can happen if you try has changed my approach too. I know that there will be many things I will never be able to do particularly well, but I also know that the approach of conductive education was a completely new approach. I bend my right knee up, I stretch my right leg out, I lift my leg up, I put my right arm down. One year ago I would have found it very difficult to do any of those things. I would also have found it very difficult to say things like forehead, nose, chin, shoulders, chest, heart, stomach, waist, finger, thumb etc. (name all parts of body). That I couldn't have done, that surprises me at my age.
>
> The weekly session also brought me to the theory that perhaps I could say this better but I know how much I am now using that I would never have said when I started with conductive education.
>
> Initially the first five minutes standing up was very painful and I

was glad that I could sit down again. At home I was sitting most of the day and never really using my legs for walking. You looked at it in a different way. You said that I should be trying to walk better every day and that I have done. To be able now to walk around the close with my walker, to actually walk half a mile up to the pub and back with the walker rather than with a wheelchair would never have been possible.

My paralysed right side is now beginning to do things and I am beginning to walk without a stick at all.

My wife is surprised by my balance now which was bad. She also knows that my breathing is so much better. I know that I had coughed week after week, now she has colds and I don't. I am reading on my own far more, of course I still get my wife to read for me to keep me up to date.

Conductive education suggests why shouldn't I read better. No one else had suggested that before and that's why I'm reading better now. I have probably said more than I should already but it simply shows

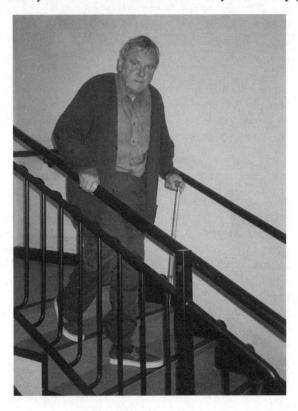

Fig. 14.4 James going down stairs

how a person can change because of a complete attempt to do things that a normal hospital would think were unnecessary or never likely to happen. This has shown for me something different.

I have been able to do a lot of movements around the house I couldn't have done. I can now go up and down the stairs. I have a lift but I try and go up and down the stairs without it as well. Gradually I have been able to spend more time walking, standing and talking to people in the close without having to sit down. Almost every time someone comes to see us they are amazed that I have changed since the last time they saw me. I think that has happened all because of the attempt of making things work that wouldn't have happened a year ago.

People talk about the work with children and this is important, but the department for the adults have very severe disabled people who get so much from the unit. The staff have made a complete difference to what it must have been 10 years ago. Once you have the mind of CE and a different way of life you won't change until you die.

I am still a very severe disabled person but my body has changed and I hope that this will continue week by week.

RUTH

Ruth was born in 1971 and shortly after birth was diagnosed with cerebral palsy quadriplegia. She attended a special school and lived at home with her mother and two sisters. At present she attends a day centre during the week and helps to run the coffee shop.

AT CONSULTATION

Ruth came to us for consultation in September 1994. At this time she was a wheelchair user and her mother lifted her in and out of her chair. She was unable to bear weight on her limbs while transferring. She could sit alone in her chair but was unable to sit without any support. Her hips were extended and so she tended to lean back in her wheelchair. She was unable to propel her wheelchair as she only had limited movement with her right hand and very little spontaneous movement with her left. At home she was able to take part in some activities but needed full care support.

The main aims for Ruth were to try and teach her how to loosen her lower limbs and begin to initiate movements with them, and to increase the use of her hands, in particular the left one. She wanted assistance so that she could play a more active role in her everyday activities. She was experiencing considerable pain in her left hip at this time.

WHAT DID RUTH ACHIEVE THROUGH CONDUCTIVE EDUCATION?

Ruth began to attend following the consultation for one session per week. Initially this was an individual session and later she was joined by another young lady with similar problems. Her placement was restricted by difficulties with funding. At present she awaits funding from Social Services, so she is being funded for the time being by a private charitable trust.

Her progress was steady and very gradual. She found it very difficult to find ways to use her limbs because she had been led to believe that they were not useful. Gradually she began to use her left hand and this enabled her to play a more active part in everyday activities, such as dressing.

At first much of Ruth's work was in a lying position because she was unable to sit securely. During the first year she was able to increase the range of movement with her lower limbs and begin to loosen the spasticity in her hips. This allowed her to learn to sit without support. She still lacks some confidence in this position, but she is able to use her hands to give her the security needed.

Much time was spent teaching Ruth how to use her arms and legs when transferring. The main aim of this was to increase her independence and also to help her mother as she was now a fully mature adult. She still needs

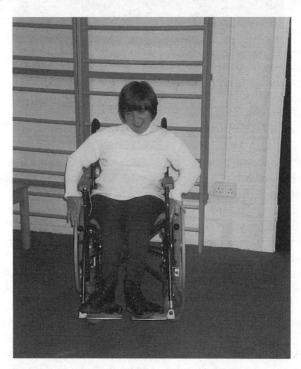

Fig. 14.5 Ruth propelling her wheelchair

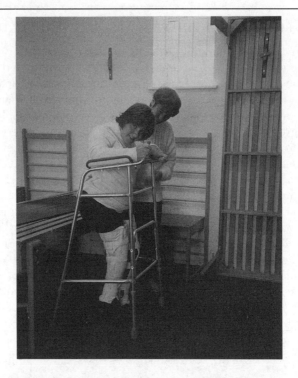

Fig. 14.6 Ruth using gaiters to stand up

help when transferring but this is only at the hips and is very gradually being reduced.

The main change was the increase in Ruth's confidence to attempt particular activities, as she proved to have tremendous determination that had gradually been lost during her childhood. This strength of character enabled her to become more active and to search for activities in which she can take part. She is able to propel her wheelchair alone for short distances. Although this is difficult, she is now able to move around when she wants to instead of being reliant on others (Figure 14.5). The pain in her hip, which she has suffered for years, has now disappeared completely.

In the last few weeks Ruth has been standing up using gaiters. She needs some help to get into a standing position, but is now able to hold this position alone for a short time. It is to be hoped that this will help her when transferring by allowing her to bear some weight through her feet. Apart from the physical aspect of standing up, it is the first time in her life that she has been able to bear weight through her own legs and this has given her a sense of purpose and achievement. She knows that she will not be able to walk any distance, but if she can bear some weight through her legs and take one or two steps then it is hoped that she will be able to learn to transfer on to the toilet and in and out of the wheelchair in a more dignified manner (Figure 14.6)

For Ruth conductive education perhaps came too late. By the time she attended her range of movement had deteriorated tremendously. The main stage of this was during adolescence when her body was growing. Again, there have been no large changes in her physical abilities, but the steps that have been made have given her a purpose, an aim and improved her own self-confidence in her abilities. These small steps have been the result of her own efforts and are very important for her. It is hoped that Ruth will continue to attend for some time to build further on these achievements.

JOHN

Born in 1927, John first began to notice that his body was shaking when he was in his mid-twenties. At this time no answers were given, and it was not until 1964 that he was diagnosed as having Parkinson's disease. He was diagnosed at a time when Levadopa was not available and John started taking a cocktail of drugs to try and control symptoms. He was directed by a doctor as to what dosages to take, which later proved to be incorrect and he nearly lost his life. In the late 1970s he was prescribed dopamine which gave him relief from his symptoms for some time.

He attended for consultation as soon as conductive education became available in the United Kingdom. For him it was 26 years after diagnosis, during which time he married, raised a family and was now 63 years of age.

AT CONSULTATION

At the time of consultation John's walking was very asymmetrical and he was unable to bend his left knee. He swung both his arms forwards and backwards when walking as if to propel himself. He lacked fine co-ordination in his right hand and had limited movement of his wrists. He was unable to stand up from a chair without pushing on the chair. His balance in standing was insecure and he found it difficult to change rhythm or direction when walking.

John's speech was very difficult to understand as the words ran into each other. He lacked gesture when conversing and very rarely took part in social conversation outside of his family. He lacked confidence when outside of his home and had tried to keep himself active with work around the house. He was taking five Sinemet per day and was experiencing some dyskinesia. He had tremor in his left hand which prevented him from carrying out some finer activities.

John had very little expectation of outcome and was unsure whether he would like the sessions. He came with an open mind to try the sessions for a few weeks – that was six years ago. He still attends regularly twice a week and hopes to continue to do so for the foreseeable future.

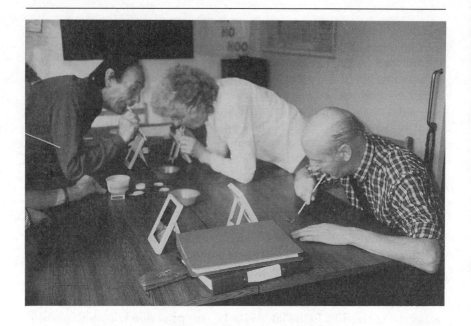

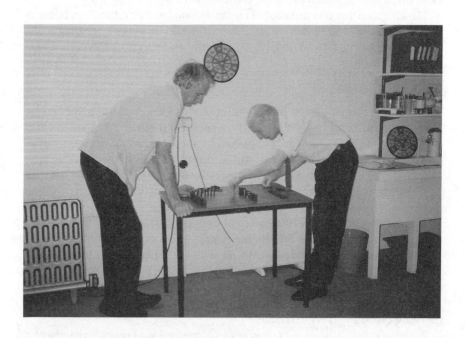

Figs. 14.7–9 (above and opposite) John joining in activities

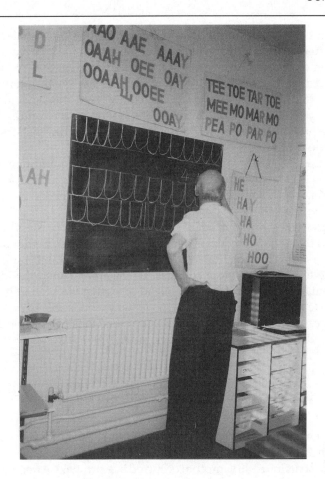

WHAT DID JOHN GAIN FROM CONDUCTIVE EDUCATION?

John began to show improvement in confidence in his own abilities, which in turn led to an increase in activity and an improvement in his movements. He found that he was able to kneel down in church and then stand up from this position, and that he was able to cross himself in church, something he had not been able to do for many years.

John is now able to deal the cards when playing, and this again has helped to increase his social confidence. He reported that people always thought he was drunk when he went to the local club because of the way that he walked. Now he is able to walk to the toilet alone, through a crowded room, with security and confidence. His writing has improved although he does not write to any great extent.

The biggest change that has happened has been the improvement in John's speech. He commented that once someone said pardon to him, when they didn't understand him, he stopped talking. He knew that there was no point in repeating what he had said because it would be even worse the second time around. His speech is now easily understood and the only thing that is left is his broad Irish accent! He has given interviews for television and radio, spoken on a chat show, read passages in front of groups of people and regularly entertains visitors to the centre. This area of change has made the greatest difference to him and has encouraged him to continue to attend.

John has attended group sessions and also had an additional speech session once a week with some other members of his group. Figures 14.7, 14.8 and 14.9 show some of the activities that he has joined in alongside his fellow group members.

John now takes three and a half to four Sinemet a day, one less than when he started the sessions six years ago. He still experiences tremor and some dyskinesia and is finding that his drugs are less predictable, but feels that he is able to cope with these changes. He has maintained the initial improvements he made and is able to lead an active life both at home and socially. He has an awareness of his movements and is able to correct them when necessary. He is able to walk outside alone for a reasonable distance. He still finds it very difficult, however, to walk and talk!

GORDON

The following is an account written by Gordon about his condition and his experience of conductive education.

> I was born in March 1943, married Betty in 1970 and have two sons born in 1972 and 1974.
>
> My first definite MS symptom occurred in April 1969. After working on a friend's car one day, I woke up the following morning without any feeling in my right hand, and very little grip. It was believed that I may have trapped a nerve in my wrist, for which I was given a course of localized heat treatment and physiotherapy. Over a period of several weeks dexterity returned, but my sense of touch is still very poor – I liken it to wearing a pair of surgical gloves.
>
> During the next seven years I suffered permanent 'pins and needles' in my feet, cold feet and lower legs. I subsequently lost all feeling in my right foot. I easily became exhausted doing comparatively simple tasks requiring effort – lifting, cutting the grass and the like. It became very difficult to walk in a straight line, especially when tired. Various visits to my then GP during this time were dismissed with 'it's all in the mind' (although I knew it wasn't) and numerous courses of Librium and Valium were prescribed which had little effect. In 1975 I was diagnosed as suffering from anxiety and depression and given antidepressants.

In June 1976 after using brilliant white emulsion paint in strong sunlight I suffered 'snow blindness' in my left eye, turning into blurred vision. I was referred to an ophthalmic consultant which subsequently led me to being admitted to hospital in September when I was diagnosed as having MS. Surprisingly, perhaps, this came as a relief as I now had a reason for my symptoms.

During the next 10 years I noticed a slow deterioration in my mobility. In 1982 my occupation as an insurance surveyor became too strenuous and I had to take a desk job with the same company. Between 1980 and 1986 I had various courses of ACTH which initially helped in the short term, but began to have less effect. I suffered two relapses within six weeks during the summer of 1987, each time being treated in hospital by methylprednisolone administered intra-venously. This was my first introduction to this steroid; after the first course I left hospital feeling able to 'shift heaven and earth', attempted to, and had a further more serious relapse.

For three days or so I lost my sense of hearing. This slowly returned, although I still have only about 20% hearing ability in my left ear. For a few days I lost all sense of balance even when sat or laid down. Co-ordination was poor. I started to use a wheelchair for all but short distances. During the next 12 months I began to feel increasingly fatigued. A desk job became an effort for longer than two hours, followed by spending the remainder of the day in bed. At meal times I was sometimes too exhausted to eat more than one course. My social life became non-existent. I finally stopped work in November 1988 on medical advice.

In July 1988 I commenced taking hyperbaric oxygen at a local ARMS centre and have continued this on a weekly basis to the present day. Although I don't notice any immediate benefit, I realize after a few days if I've missed a session. This could be psychological of course.

My condition then stabilized and slightly improved. However, in the summer of 1992 I had a further relapse after suffering a trauma. This caused very severe fatigue and poor co-ordination. I was advised to rest, and after five months returned almost to my pre-trauma condition without any medication. During this time I had continued weekly hyperbaric oxygen and light physiotherapy. I also heard of conductive education from a fellow sufferer who had found it bene-ficial.

Early in 1993 I attended an initial consultation and was sub-sequently offered a place on a six-week course followed by a further course of similar duration. On each course I attended for two hours twice weekly. To begin with I found conductive education extremely tiring. I was exhausted after a two-hour session, and some I found were more difficult and tiring than others. However, during the second course I became more able to cope with this problem and I can now manage courses attending each day for two or three weeks.

I find this type of course more beneficial than once or twice a week over a longer period. The intensity improves my stamina and co-ordination which I can then maintain for four to five months.

I was told on my initial consultation that I had deteriorated over almost 20 years and that I must not expect immediate improvements. This is true; it has taken almost three years to incorporate lessons and routines learnt into daily life without thinking. Having now achieved this, I find simple things like washing and dressing, sitting and standing are all now easier. This in turn means I am generally less fatigued and enjoy a better quality of life.

Gordon still continues to attend two or three courses during a 12-month period. He has been able not only to maintain his movements but to use techniques which make these easier.

SAMANTHA

The following is an account written by Samantha following several trips to the Petö Institute and to the National Institute in Birmingham. She was born in 1959 and diagnosed as having MS in 1988.

I was first introduced to conductive education in 1992 when I was fortunate enough to attend the Petö Institute in Budapest. I had no real expectations, but was delighted to find that my mobility, and ability to walk fairly long distances improved considerably over the three-week period. I think the overriding factor was the optimism and positive attitude of the conductors.

When I first arrived for consultation I met Agi, who took my walking stick and implied that I didn't really need it! In fact at that time I probably didn't need it, and soon began to walk everywhere completely unaided. I think the most important element was that other people believed in my capabilities, and I soon began to think that if other people thought I could do it – then maybe I could! My confidence increased tremendously, but the nature of the illness being what it is, I soon began to suffer relapses.

I travelled to Hungary twice in the subsequent years and each time felt as though I had improved considerably. I was therefore delighted to hear that a centre for conductive education was being established in Birmingham. This cut down considerably the cost of obtaining this specialized therapy, especially as I was able to stay with my 'in-laws'! I find the programme virtually the same as in Hungary, with the added benefit of English being spoken. I think that cost is prohibitive for most people who have to find accommodation.

When Samantha arrived in January 1994 her movements were very limited due to several relapses in her condition. She needed a stick when walking, her balance was poor and there was severe spasticity in her right leg. She again showed improvement over the space of the course and is able to maintain this improvement for about three months, following which she attends another course.

Although her condition has gradually deteriorated over the past few years, Samantha is still able to walk and live an active life at home. Over the months between visits she tends to lose some of her movements but usually returns to her previous level following a few sessions. She goes on to say:

> I think one of the major benefits is reaching some understanding of the way the therapy works. I find that the movements used in the sessions are used in everyday living – stretching to reach something from a shelf, bending to pick something up from the floor, etc. I have found that I can cope very well alone in the house but still haven't achieved enough confidence to venture out on my own.
>
> I really think I have benefited from conductive education, if only because of the level of exercise involved. I do know, however, that a high degree of independence can be achieved and maintained by regular visits to Birmingham.

STEPHEN

Stephen, a journalist, was born in 1958 and in 1984 was involved in a road traffic accident which left him with damage to the brain stem. This left him with very little movement, no speech for one year and an intact intellect.

He first came to the Institute in 1992 but at this time there was no regular provision available for him. He was given a programme to work on at home but this was very limited. In 1993 the Institute was able to expand its work and Stephen started to attend regularly. He has attended once a week since, with his father bringing him by car from Aylesbury to Birmingham for the session.

AT CONSULTATION

In 1992 when Stephen first attended he was able to stand in a standing frame, which he did for at least one hour a day. He used an electric wheelchair around the house and required full-time care from his wife and professional carers.

When sitting in his chair Stephen leant to the right and his head was bent forward. At this time he had reduced control of his neck and used to wear a neck collar when travelling to prevent his head falling forward. He had limited use of his hands and his elbows were held flexed. His right hand was held in a fist and he was unable to bend the fingers of his left hand due to an earlier operation to extend his fingers.

When performing a movement, the whole of Stephen's body moved. He was unable to isolate movements and this made it very difficult to balance in a sitting position. He was able to speak but articulation was very poor and there was limited volume. His breathing technique was very shallow and this hindered his speech. When lying down he was unable to relax his head back towards the bed and had to lie with his shoulders in a raised position.

Our aims, which were set with Stephen, were to try and increase his overall range of movement, particularly on the right side, to improve his articulation and breathing, to teach him to stand with minimal help and to take a few steps with support. In order to achieve these, we first had to teach him how to reduce his spasticity and how to initiate movements from different parts of the body.

WHAT SUCCESS DID STEPHEN FIND THROUGH CONDUCTIVE EDUCATION?

Stephen had severe spasticity so this process took a long time. In 1996, however, he is able to stand up in parallel bars or at wall bars for a short time alone; he is able to take steps in the bars requiring only minimal assistance with transferring his weight. His volume of speech has improved as has his breathing technique. His articulation is still poor but his speech can now be understood more easily.

Stephen is able to isolate movements, giving him greater control over his body. The movements in his upper limbs have improved and, although his neck is still a little stiff, he is able to loosen this and no longer uses a collar when travelling. He is able to sit without support and maintain his balance when moving his upper limbs. His finer movements, although still difficult, have improved.

Stephen has two young children at home and is able to play a more active role as a father. He still needs carers to help him with daily activities but he is able to take a more active role. He has wall bars at home and is able to stand at these during the day. The progress Stephen has made has been slow and gradual, but each step has been a huge achievement for him. The following is a summary of his thoughts on his progress during the last three years.

First heard of this 'new' method of treating brain injuries purely from a magazine article. But asking around it seemed that no doctors or nurses in a large general hospital had a clue of the best way to treat a head injury like mine. All the doctors and nurses could just see my muscles stiffening up to the point of no return. After three years conductive education, I have achieved a lot more than I could possibly have hoped to see with traditional physiotherapy. It has also assisted me to move myself and position any part or my whole body comfortably on the plinth for work to even begin.

In fact it is vital, as one conductor explained to me, to be able to get the correct position to even begin an exercise as relaxed and comfortable as possible. Then, just a little more effort is required to achieve the required movement. It is here that I have had particular trouble lately, finding the correct level of effort to make the movement without making greatly exaggerated movements. This will help me find and maintain my position of balance. Just lifting my leg, by moving only my foot, was terribly difficult for some time. And I still have terrible trouble isolating the position of my head and neck when performing some totally unconnected movements. Being able to complete certain tasks without any assistance has been successfully achieved.

It has been made clear to me that it is much better and more comfortable to get into a standing position from time to time. Just being able to get up out of a sitting position took a lot of effort initially, but it can now be achieved quite simply and quickly. Just transferring the whole body from one place to another in comfort and quickly takes a lot of knowledge and experience and this is one aspect the

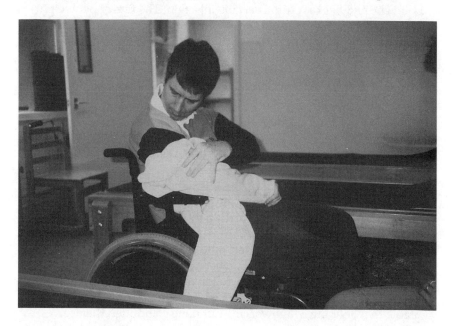

Fig. 14.10 Stephen putting on his jumper

conductors have instilled right from the beginning. They seem to know just which bits to move and by how much.

It is hoped that Stephen will continue to show stages of improvement. His movements will always remain a challenge but we hope to give him some techniques to make them a little easier.

Below is a photograph of Stephen putting on his own jumper (Figure 14.10). These types of activity allow the individual to apply the tasks they have been learning to an everyday situation. This is where the emphasis of conductive education is placed.

RACHEL

Rachel was born in 1969 and first came to our institute in November 1995. She was the victim of vaccine damage in childhood and as a result has very severe disabilities.

RACHEL'S HISTORY

The following is an account, written by her mother, of Rachel's difficulties.

Rachel was born, after a normal pregnancy, weighing 7lbs 10oz. She was breast-fed and gained 8lbs 6ozs in the first six months, at which point she had her first triple vaccine injection. The rate of her weight gain dropped to 3lbs 14oz in the next six months and to 2lbs 11oz in the following year. From the age of four years to eight years she actually lost weight.

During the first six months of her life she made normal progress which was confirmed by the clinic at which she regularly attended. She would in those early months hold a rusk and feed herself with it, but following the injections her progress slowed and eventually stopped.

At nine months she was not sitting up so professional advice was sought; assurances were given that nothing was wrong and that the only problem was slow muscle development; the opinion expressed was that with time this would improve. As no diagnosis of her condition was given to us, eventually a further opinion was requested and we were referred to Great Ormond Street Hospital, London.

There, many tests were carried out and, as a result, we were informed that various conditions had been eliminated but no consultant would offer a positive opinion as to the real cause of her retardation. On many occasions we asked whether her condition could be attributable to whooping cough vaccine but none committed themselves.

In 1977 an approach was made to us by a friend who after qualifying as a Doctor in Czechoslovakia, came to England and, after obtaining an MSc. at Manchester University took up research at the National Institute at Mill Hill, London. At this time research was being carried out into the effects of the whooping cough vaccine. After carrying out tests on many samples of Rachel's urine, it was found that substances which should have gone into muscle, nerve and bone development were passing through her system, all as a result of the effect of the vaccine. Rachel's condition was so severe at that time that fears were expressed for her survival, but after a course of a proprietary product, Keetavite, containing Biotin, her condition gradually improved and she began to gain weight.

Since that time her general health has improved wonderfully but she has been unable to feed herself and all her food has to be mashed. Everything in the way of dressing, washing etc. has to be done for her. The severe curvature of her spine causes her pain and has added to her problems.

WHAT COULD CONDUCTIVE EDUCATION DO FOR RACHEL?

When Rachel came to us we were unsure if we would be able to offer any help. We had not previously worked with people suffering vaccine damage and were unsure of any benefits to be gained. This was discussed with her parents and we all decided that we would never know unless we gave Rachel a chance and that she would make that final decision by her reaction to the sessions.

Although Rachel has no verbal communication, she is able to show her feelings, whether these be pain, happiness or displeasure. Initially her mother worked alongside her guided by a conductor and, as we gradually were able to develop a rapport with Rachel, it was decided that she would be able to work alone.

Rachel obviously enjoys the sessions, and having learnt what is expected of her she is now able to perform a number of movements with minimal assistance from us. The biggest change we have noticed is that she now has eye contact with us and is showing interest in her surroundings. Her walking has improved and she is more able to lift her feet. The constant pain that she was suffering from her spine appears to have lessened and this has given her greater freedom.

Her mother reports:

After hearing of a limited development of conductive education in Coventry, the National Institute was contacted and, following an assessment, Rachel commenced individual sessions at the National Institute in Birmingham at the beginning of November 1995. We feel that the warm and patient approach of the staff has been most helpful in gaining her confidence. She obviously had severe inhibitions after so much frustration, but her walking is improved through the expert guidance and we find her muscles are generally more relaxed, which means that she can mount the stairs more easily though still needing assistance. Her eye contact is improving as also are her toileting and drinking. We feel that the fact that Rachel realizes that an attempt is being made to improve the quality of her life has given her real encouragement and for the most part she is cheerful and takes more interest in her surroundings.

Whilst Rachel's improvements will be limited physically, she will continue to attend the Institute until it is felt that she is no longer showing any benefit. Apart from the sessions at the Institute and day centre provision, Rachel has no other provision to stimulate her physically or intellectually. Her parents have had to carry that role over the years and it is due to their dedication, love and untiring work for their daughter that she is beginning to show the signs of progress we have seen over the past year.

Figure 14.11 below shows Rachel walking.

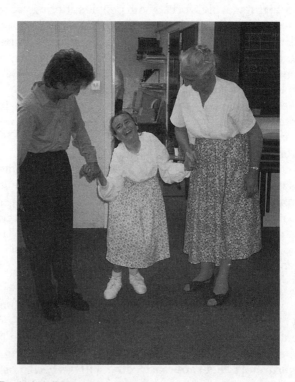

Fig. 14.11 Rachel walking

JEFF

Jeff was born in 1947 and ran his own business. In July 1993 he was suffering from a severe sore throat which, following a series of problems, led to anoxia. He was hospitalized and on a ventilator for two weeks. It took another three months for what is described as a gradual awakening. He was left with a severe visual problem, speech problem and extensive physical disabilities. His intellect remained intact as did his memory.

HOW DID CONDUCTIVE EDUCATION HELP JEFF?

Jeff first came to the Institute in January 1995 for a three-week course. He attended daily for 15 sessions and stayed in a hotel with his wife for the duration of the course. His movements were very ataxic and he was unable to walk without holding on to someone for balance. His upper limbs had spasticity, the left one being more severe. His overall movements were slow and he was unable to sit up with stretched legs alone.

Jeff's face lacked expression and his speech was slow and scanting. He had a tic from his right shoulder up to his head. Following his blindness some sight had returned, but he was only able to see outlines and had double vision. He found it difficult to turn over in bed, do up buttons and needed a great deal of care from his wife and was unable to work.

Following the three-week course Jeff had shown improvement in a number of areas. Firstly his self-confidence increased so he was able to walk alone with reasonable security, he was able to swing his arms a little when walking and his style was generally more relaxed. He was able to bend his knees slightly when stepping and this allowed him to use the whole of his foot when walking, thus enabling him to successfully transfer the weight from one foot to the other. His spacial awareness increased so he was more able to find and maintain a symmetrical position.

The co-ordination and flexibility of Jeff's hand movements increased and, although still showing signs of spasticity, he was more able to perform fine movements. The rhythm of his movements increased and, although these were still a little slow, much of this was due to hesitation from lack of visual field. His tic more or less disappeared and was only noticeable when he was very tired.

WHAT WAS JEFF'S EXPERIENCE OF CONDUCTIVE EDUCATION?

Using a talking computer Jeff wrote about his own experience during those three weeks.

I learnt about conductive education through my wife reading a news item a few years ago. She recalled this when the end of my NHS treatment came and, in short, I was left to my own devices. I suppose that we were looking for a more definite type of 'hands on' treatment and so were prepared to try anything. My wife wrote to the Pető Institute in Budapest and we received an appointment to go there a few months later. Then, by chance, a friend of ours living a few doors down the road mentioned our proposed trip to his neighbour whose job is to distribute charity monies given by The Ford Motor Company. This chap said that he had sent some funds to a charity of the same name in the Cardiff area and we immediately contacted that organization. By chance there was a conductor there at the time, but only for another few days. So we hurriedly drove to South Wales for me to be assessed by this lady conductor.

(This centre was only able to take children with cerebral palsy, so a contact was made with The National Institute and Jeff was then given a placement at Birmingham for a few weeks later.)

When I first started I thought the exercises were a little too simple and I could not see how conductive education could possibly help my problems. In fact, after the first week I decided not to return for the remaining fortnight's sessions. But then I thought, what the hell, I might as well sit here in sunny Brum as anywhere else!

In the second week I found the confidence to begin walking on my own. Up to then I had relied on someone holding on to me. This of course was a major breakthrough for me. Although I was still afraid to take many steps alone, this has gradually abated and the confidence grown to such an extent that I can now walk around my house alone with total confidence.

This of course means that I *never* use my wheelchair now. You can imagine what that means to me and, of course, everyone else in my family. No more lugging the heavy thing around, damaging the car or breaking people's backs. Not using the wheelchair has also got me a great deal fitter and of course more mobile when going into restaurants, cinemas and shops. The effect on my family has been tremendous, with my wife winning the greater amount since she took the brunt of the load before I walked on my own.

Jeff still continues to show improvement but unfortunately has been unable to attend for any further courses, due to the financial restrictions of accommodation and fees for attending. His sight is still very poor, but both he and his wife are determined to continue to work with this. Maybe if conductive education becomes more readily available with statutory funding, then Jeff and others in his situation would be able to reap the benefits on a longer term.

Questions and answers

15

PROVISION OF CONDUCTIVE EDUCATION

Is conductive education available from the National Health Service or through social services?

At present it is very difficult to gain any public funding or provision for conductive education. There are isolated cases where GPs may fund an individual within their practice. Social services throughout the country do fund places for adults, but these are decided on an individual basis.

Whilst statutory funding for services is difficult to obtain the climate is beginning to change. Public services are now obliged to consider services from the private sector, therefore statutory funding should always be considered.

SUITABILITY OF CONDUCTIVE EDUCATION

Who is suitable for conductive education?

This is a very common question. Perhaps it should be turned around and we should ask who is conductive education suitable for.

Generally, but not exclusively, conductive education is a system of education for people with neurological disorders. The system itself, as with other forms of education, will be more suitable for some people than others. This however, does not depend on the system but on the person receiving it. Each individual consultation will aim to set realistic goals and the ways of achieving these should be explained to the individual, who is then able to decide whether they wish to pursue this course or not.

Each individual will gain something different, and the conductor cannot stand in judgement as to the extent of this gain or importance of this gain for the person. We would suggest that each individual is given a trial period, and during the course they can find out for themselves whether they find the system beneficial. If progress is reviewed and monitored regularly then the individual will be in a position to discuss the benefits and decide whether the system is appropriate for them.

MUSIC

Does conductive education use music?

One of the myths of conductive education is that it is music-based. With children, music, rhythms and songs are regularly used as with any other forms of education, and music plays a role in the National Curriculum.

In Hungary music has a very important role within the curriculum, and children learn a specific repertoire of songs during their schooling. Thus one may expect to hear music and singing when in Hungary. In the United Kingdom music plays the same role. For many children a song or rhyme will help to complete the activity and make it enjoyable. For adults, music is rarely used.

The strong use of rhythm should not be confused with the use of music. The rhythm is used to assist the teaching of motor skill, music is used for enjoyment. The two may be combined but, generally, adults with motor disorders find it very difficult to concentrate on a number of skills at any one time. Singing may detract from walking or from other movement skills, but on the other hand singing may increase lung capacity and can help with speech.

Although music can play a role in conductive education, it is not an integral part of the system, but the rhythm of movement is an essential part of the whole system. Our bodies do not move naturally in a musical rhythm; if we want to increase the level of motor skill then we have to teach rhythm, not music.

AN INTENSIVE SYSTEM

Conductive education is often described as an intensive system. Does this mean that exercises must be carried out every day?

Firstly, it is important to draw a distinction between exercises and the tasks of conductive education. The tasks used are the teaching medium for everyday living skills. If a person wishes to practise particular tasks, then they may find that their level of skill improves. Tasks are not designed to exercise muscles but to teach strategies for performing skills. If these strategies are not practised in context then they will have no meaning and will not be useful skills.

An average person is awake and active for around 14 to 16 hours a day. If that person is taught how to use the movement skills they have learnt, then they will be using these skills for this amount of time. If they perform exercises, then it is likely that they will do this for one or two hours a day and then forget about it. The tasks learnt have to be incorporated into daily life if they are to be useful, and they may need to be practised until the person is able to use them. If they are aware of their own abilities then they can begin to build these tasks into everyday life.

Learning only begins when this process starts. The conductor uses the task series as a teacher may use the blackboard. Tasks are only a medium for teaching, they do not have to be learnt in the format they are taught, but the skill has to be generalized and used in all situations throughout the day.

OTHER THERAPIES

Is it possible to attend other therapy sessions alongside conductive education?

Yes. It is very important that each individual receives as much help as they can in overcoming their difficulties. Contrary to popular belief, other therapies will not affect conductive education, just as conductive education will not affect other therapies. Each individual should have access to as many different systems and therapies as possible, as this will enable them to find the ones that most suit their needs.

Each one of us uses our body in a different way. If we have a neurological condition that affects movement, then we need to gain as much experience as we can. Conductive education is teaching how to use motor skills and this cannot be contradicted by any other form of treatment. Service users should be actively encouraged to use all the services available to them.

ADULT CONDUCTIVE EDUCATION

Conductive education is always shown as being available for children with cerebral palsy. Does this mean that it is for children and has been adapted for adults?

It is true that the media usually show conductive education in relation to children with cerebral palsy and that the main provision within the United Kingdom is for this group. Conductive Education, however, began with adults. There is evidence to suggest that adults with Parkinson's disease have been attending conductive education in Hungary since the 1960s.

Conductive education is, as its name suggests, an educational system.

There is no such thing as an education for children alone. Adults also benefit from education, and it is up to the conductor to ensure that the methods of teaching used are appropriate for adults. The system itself is neither for children nor adults; it is an educational approach.

CONDUCTIVE EDUCATION AND DIAGNOSIS

Does it matter how long ago a person was diagnosed?

Generally this does not matter, but it will depend on the diagnosis of the individual. For someone with Parkinson's disease or multiple sclerosis, the length of diagnosis is not a contributing factor. For those with cerebral palsy, whilst the age of the person does not preclude them from a service, there will naturally be smaller steps of improvement than with a young child. Head injuries and strokes are also within this category, as we know that progress slows down about two years after the accident or stroke.

However, it is important to emphasize that any small steps of improvement made will have a beneficial effect on the everyday life of the individual, and these steps should not be underestimated. Any adult can continue to learn throughout their life span, and the same is true of those with a neurological condition. In order to achieve this, however, there must be an input. Therefore the length of time since diagnosis is not important but the individual concerned must realize that progress will be made in small stages that may take some time to achieve. This should not be used as an excuse for not providing for people; learning will still take place.

COUNTING

Do adults have to count? They often feel very self-conscious when doing this.

Counting is used to help to teach the rhythm of movements. It plays a very important role. Counting out loud is a teaching tool for the conductor as it enables them to monitor the whole group. In addition, verbal speech helps with breathing technique and requires that the person concentrate on more than one thing at a time.

How many times do we move or speak? Usually the two are combined. It is not essential that the adult counts out loud if they feel that this is embarrassing or detracts from their ability to join in a group. In this case they should be encouraged to count to themselves quietly. The importance of counting should be clearly explained to them. In some groups verbal counting actually assists performance.

The conductor must give the explanations to the individual and establish a setting where the person feels comfortable. Usually adults will feel self-conscious if they are unable to see the relevance of what they are being asked to do; a good explanation often helps this situation.

CONDUCTIVE EDUCATION IS MORE THAN EXERCISE

I use these exercises with my patients already. What else can conductive education offer?

As already mentioned above, the tasks of conductive education should not be seen as exercises. Naturally any professional who is working in the field of movement will use the same movements. Our bodies can only produce a limited number of movements. The way we use these movements is more important than the movement itself.

Conductive education does not teach the movement but motor skill, and in order to do this certain movements will need to be taught. Exercise classes, therapy sessions and individual exercise programmes will all use the same movements; it is the reason for using these that will differ. One may attend an exercise class to improve flexibility, increase muscle strength or improve level of motor skill. The tasks are also used alongside a complete educational system and are only one part of the whole system.

WALKING

I have heard that conductive education places an emphasis on walking. Does this mean that only someone who has the capacity to walk will benefit?

Unfortunately media coverage usually places an emphasis on walking as this is of greatest interest to the reader or viewer. Conductive education aims to teach motor skills as applicable to the individual person. It is possible that walking may not be a priority for an individual or that it is too high a goal to aim for.

The aims in conductive education have to be placed at a realistic level. They should be set in consultation with the individual concerned and reflect their personal needs. Walking is only a priority if it is a realistic goal and if the individual themselves places an emphasis on it in order to improve their everyday living skills.

GROUP WORK

Not everyone likes to work within a group. Does conductive education only take place in groups?

Generally, in education, it is reported that groups are beneficial to learning. For this reason conductive education often takes place within groups.

These groups must be carefully constructed and the conductor has to work with the group as a whole.

At times individual sessions may also take place, and there are a number of circumstances where these sessions may be of more benefit. If the individual themselves requests that they only wish individual sessions, the conductor will introduce them to a group if possible and encourage them to work with a group, but the final decision is left to the individual concerned.

There are times where a group may not meet the needs of an individual. This is particularly true if the centre has limited resources. Individuals should only be placed in groups that will meet their needs. If there is a limit to the number of groups then the person may need to work as an individual. It is possible that an individual will work on their own for a few sessions and then join a group. There are also situations where the person may receive a service within their own home, and this is usually on an individual basis. Whilst group-work is preferable as it provides a positive environment and members can share experiences and knowledge, there are times when an individual session will best meet the needs of that person.

AVAILABILITY OF CONDUCTIVE EDUCATION

Where is conductive education for adults available?

Unfortunately there is still a limited provision for adults within the United Kingdom, the majority of which is fairly scattered. Provision is continually changing and therefore it is not appropriate to list the places where it is available. Information about centres is available from the National Library of Conductive Education in Birmingham, and the Parkinson's Disease Society often have access to centres running courses as do SCOPE and the Stroke Association. In addition, the United Kingdom Federation for Conductive Education, based in London, will have access to information and centres that are members of their organization. Provision is increasing, and each person should contact any organization concerned with conductive education to receive an up-to-date list of centres running courses for adults.

ATTENDANCE AT SESSIONS

How long should each individual attend sessions for?

Conductive education is not a treatment and therefore does not have timed courses. Each individual will find that the length of benefit varies.

In general, a person should attend for at least 15 sessions initially as this will give them time to gain an insight into the benefits for them. This should then be followed up. Any progressive condition will need to be monitored on a regular basis for as long as that person is able to receive some benefit. For non-progressive conditions, the person should continue to attend as long as they feel they are able to achieve the goals set and that these goals are appropriate.

Appendix

Questionnaire completed by participants suffering from Parkinson's disease. Each participant scored their own abilities on a scale of 1 to 7, where 7 indicated without difficulty and 1 with extreme difficulty.

SECTION 1 LYING POSITION

1. Sleeping
2. Getting into bed
3. Getting out of bed
4. Turning over in bed

SECTION 2 SITTING

1. Sitting up
2. Sitting
3. Sitting down

SECTION 3 STANDING

1. Weight bearing
2. Standing up
3. Stability of standing
4. Starting to move
5. Stopping
6. Coming out of enclosed space
7. Opening the door, going through and closing door
8. Walking with help
9. Walking without help
10. Walking at home
11. Walking in the street

12. Walking around other people
13. Walking short distances
14. Walking on an uneven surface
15. Walking through a crowd
16. Use of public transport
17. Crouching down
18. Kneeling
19. Standing up from the floor
20. Lifting arms above head

SECTION 4 SPEECH, READING, WRITING, MEMORY

1. Initiating speech
2. Volume of speech
3. Clarity of speech
4. Intonation – variation
5. Use of mimicry when talking
6. Use of gestures when talking
7. Use of gestures without speech, e.g. smiling, raising eyebrows, etc.
8. Talking on the telephone
9. Confidence in making contact with other people
10. Talking to unfamiliar people, e.g. speeches, lectures, etc.
11. Silent reading
12. Reading out loud
13. Retelling a story
14. Short-term memory
15. Long-term memory
16. Breathing capacity – short, superficial, optimal, long
17. Signature
18. Writing a postcard
19. Writing a letter
20. Writing with a typewriter/word processor

SECTION 5 BATHING

1. Drying with a towel
2. Shaving
3. Washing hair
4. Drying hair
5. Brushing or combing hair

SECTION 6 DRESSING AND UNDRESSING

1. Top clothes
2. Underwear
3. Shoes
4. Buttoning
5. Tying laces
6. Knotting
7. Poppers/press studs
8. Velcro
9. Zip
10. Tie
11. Doing a buckle
12. Doing up a belt

SECTION 7 EATING

1. Laying the table
2. Serving from a dish
3. Use of knife
4. Use of fork
5. Use of spoon
6. Drinking with a handled cup
7. Drinking with a glass

SECTION 8 SELF-HELP SKILLS

1. Shopping
2. Washing
3. Wringing clothes
4. Ironing
5. Doing odd jobs
6. Use of tools
7. Climbing a ladder
8. Use of scissors
9. Driving
10. Manipulating small coins

References and further reading

Ashburn, D. and De Souza, L. (1988) An approach to the management of multiple sclerosis. *Physiotherapy Practice*, **4**, 139–45.

Bairstow, P., Cochrane, R. and Rusk, I. (1991) Selection of children with cerebral palsy for conductive education and the characteristics of children judged suitable and unsuitable. *Developmental Medicine and Child Neurology*, **33**, 984–92.

Baker, M. (1985) Report on a visit to Petö Institute, Hungary, 25 March–1 April 1985. Unpublished paper held at National Library for Conductive Education, Birmingham.

Baldwin, S. (1993) *The Myth of Community Care: An Alternative Neighbourhood Model of Care*, Chapman & Hall, London.

Banks, Moira A. (ed.) (1986) *Stroke*, Churchill Livingstone, New York.

Beck, A.T., Ward, C.H. *et al.* (1964) An inventory for measuring depression. *Arch. Gen. Psychiatry* **4**, 561–71

Birdwood, G.F.B., Gilder, S.S.B. and Wink, C.A.S. (1971) *Parkinson's Disease. A New Approach to Treatment*, Academic Press, London.

Blaxter, M. (1980) *The Meaning of Disability*, Heinmann Educational Books Ltd, London.

Bleck, E. (1987) *Orthopaedic Management in Cerebral Palsy*, Blackwell Scientific Publications Ltd, Oxford.

Bornat, J., Pereira, C., Pilgrim, D. *et al.* (1993) *Community Care: A Reader*, Macmillan in association with Open University.

Brechin, A., Liddiard, P. and Swain, J. (1983) *Handicap in a Social World*, 2nd edn, for Open University, Hodder & Stoughton Ltd, Kent.

Caird, F. (1991) *Rehabilitation in Parkinson's Disease*, Chapman & Hall, London.

Clifford Rose, F. and Capildeo, R. (1981) *STROKE. The Facts*, Oxford University Press, Oxford.

Cornell, S. (1996) *The Complete MS Body Manual*, Under Pressure Publications, Chelmsford.

Cottam, P. and Sutton, A. (1986) *Conductive Education. A System for Overcoming Motor Disorder*, Croom Helm, London.

Cotton, E. and Kinsman, R. (1983) *Conductive Education for Adult Hemiplegia*, Churchill Livingstone, Edinburgh.

Crompton, S. (1988) Standing on their own two feet. *Nursing Times*, 9 November, Vol. 84, No. 45.

Davidson, R. and Hunter, S. (1994) *Community Care in Practice*, B.T.Bashford Ltd, London.

De Souza, L. (1990) *Multiple Sclerosis. Approaches to management*, Chapman & Hall, London.

Dorros, S. (1981) *Parkinson's: A Patient's View*, Seven Locks Press, Washington D.C.

Duncan, Pamela W. and Badke, Mary Beth (1987) *STROKE REHABILITATION. The Recovery of Motor Control*, Year Book Medical Publishers, Inc., Chicago.

Fahn, S. and Elton, R.L. (1987) Unified Parkinson's Disease Rating Scale, in Fahn, S. and Marsden, C.D. (eds), *Recent Developments in Parkinson's Disease, Vol. 2*, pp. 153–64. Florahm Park, NJ, Macmillan Health Care Information.

Finley, L.J. and Capiledo, R. (1984) *Movement Disorders: Tremor*, Macmillan Press Ltd, London.

Forsythe, E. (1988) *Multiple Sclerois. Exploring Sickness and Health*, Faber & Faber Ltd, London.

Franklyn, S. (1979) Physiotherapy techniques and Parkinson's disease. Unpublished paper held at National Library for Conductive Education, Birmingham.

Fussey, I. and Giles, G.M. (1988) *Rehabilitation of the Severely Brain Injured Adult: A practical approach*, Croom Helm, London.

Garner, R. (1990) *Acute Head Injury. Practical management in rehabilitation*. Chapman & Hall, London.

Gibberd, F.B. and Kinnear, E. (1981) Controlled trial of physiotherapy and occupational therapy for Parkinson's disease. *British Medical Journal*, **282**, 1196.

Giles, G.M. and Clark-Wilson, J. (1993) *Brain Injury Rehabilitation. A neurofunctional approach*, Chapman & Hall, London.

Godwin-Austen, Dr R. (1984) *The Parkinson's Disease Handbook*, W.W.Norton & Company. New York and London.

Goodall, C. (1993) Stroke and conductive education. *Abilities*, Fall 1993, p 81.

Griffiths, M. and Clegg, M. (1988) *Cerebral Palsy: Problems and Practice*, Human Horizon Series. Souvenir Press, London.

Hancock, R. and Jarvis, C. (1994) *The long term effects of being a carer*, HMSO.

Hári, M. (1984) Conductive education. Unpublished paper held at National Library for Conductive Education, Birmingham.

Hári, M. (1990) The History of Conductive Education and the Educational Principles of the Petö System. Unpublished paper presented at World Congress, Budapest, 1990. Held at National Library for Conductive Education, Birmingham.

Hári, M and Akos, K. (1988) *Conductive Education*, Tavistock/Routledge.

Haug, G. (ed.) (1991) *Dina. A mother practises Conductive Education*, Foundation for Conductive Education, Birmingham.

Hayward, L. (1985) M.S. at the Petö Institute. Unpublished paper held at National Library for Conductive Education, Birmingham.

HMSO (1990) *National Health Service and Community Care Act*.

Hoehn, M.M. and Yahr, M.D. (1967) Parkinsonism: onset, progression and mortality. *Neurology*, **17**, 427–42.

Howard, R. and Verrier, M. (1989) Conductive education approach for retraining motor performance in patients with long-standing hemiparesis: case studies. *Physiotherapy Canada*, vol. 41, no. 4, pp. 204–8

Ingram, T.T.S., Jameson, S., Errington, J. *et al.* (1964) *Living with Cerebral Palsy*, Clinics in Developmental Medicine No. 14, Heinemann Medical Books Ltd, London.

International Petö Foundation (1989) *Training leaflet*, Petö Institute, Budapest.

Jacobs, L., O'Malley, J., Freeman, A. *et al.* (1981) Intrathecal interferon reduces exacerbations of multiple sclerosis. *Science*, **214**, 1026–28.

Kinsman, R. (1987) When the team fails, the conductor may succeed. *Geriatric Medicine*, September, pp. 62–6.

Kinsman, R. *et al.* (1988) A conductive education approach for adults with neurological dysfunction. *Physiotherapy*, vol. 74, no. 5, p. 227.

Leighton, J.P. (1972). *The Principles and Practice of Youth and Community Work*, Chester House Publications, London.

Levitt, S. (1982) *Treatment of Cerebral Palsy and Motor Delay*, 2nd edn. Blackwell Scientific Publications, Oxford.

Lubbock, G. (ed.) (1983) *Stroke Care: An Interdisciplinary Approach*, Faber and Faber, London.

Luria, A.R. (1973) *The Working Brain. An Introduction to Neuropsychology*,. Penguin Books Ltd, London.

Matthews, W.B., Acheson, E.D., Batchelor, J.R. *et al.* (eds) (1985) *McAlpine's Multiple Sclerosis*, Churchill Livingstone, London.

McAlpine, D. (1972) *Multiple Sclerosis: a reappraisal*, Churchill Livingstone, Edinburgh.

McGoon, D.C. (1990) *The Parkinson's Handbook*, W.W. Norton & Company, New York.

McKinlay, M. (1990) Conductive Education in Hungary and Britain. *Health Visitor*, vol. 63, No. 9.

Mulley, G.P. (1988) *Practical Management of Stroke*, Chapman & Hall, London.

Multiple Sclerosis Society (1990) *An Information Pack for Professional Carers*, H & M Printing Co.

Multiple Sclerosis Society (1995) *Multiple Sclerosis and Beta Interferon. What the charities say. A guide for people with MS, their families and carers.*

Murdoch, B.E. (1992) *Acquired Speech and Language Disorders*, Chapman & Hall, London.

Nanton, V. (1984) Verbal Regulation. Conductive education and Parkinson's disease. Unpublished paper held at National Library for Conductive Education, Birmingham.

Nanton, V. (1985) Psychological intervention in Parkinson's disease. Unpublished paper held at National Library for Conductive Education, Birmingham.

Nappi, G. and Caraceni, T. (1989) *Parkinsonism: Diagnosis and treatment*, Laurel House Publishing Co., Inc., USA.

Olanow, C.W. and Lieberman, A.N. (1992) *The Scientific Basis for the Treatment of Parkinson's Disease*, The Parthenon Publishing Group. Lancs., UK.

Oxtoby, M. and Wiliams, A. (1995) *Parkinson's At Your Fingertips*, Class Publishing, London.

Parkinson's Disease Society. *The Drug Treatment of Parkinson's Disease*, general publication.

Parkinson, J. (1992) An essay on the shaking palsy. Macmillan Magazines Ltd.

Pentland, B. (1987) The effects of reduced expression in Parkinson's disease on impression formation by health professionals. *Clinical Rehabilitation*. vol. 1, pp. 307–13.

Poser, C. (1984) *Diagnosis of Multiple Sclerosis*, Thieme Stratton Inc., New York.

Povey, R., Dowie, R. and Prett, G. (1981) *Learning to Live with Multiple Sclerosis*, Sheldon Press, London.

Read, J. (1988) *Come Wind, Come Weather*, 2nd edn. Foundation for Conductive Education, Birmingham.

Rinne, U.K., Klinger, M. and Stamm, G. (1980) *Parkinson's disease. Current progress, problems and management*. Proceedings of Northern European Symposium on PD, Helsinki, Nov. 6–8, Elsevier, North-Holland Biomedical Press.

Rosenthal, M., Griffith, E.R., Bond, M.R. *et al.* (1990) *Rehabilitation of the adult and child with traumatic brain injury*, 2nd ed, F.A. Davis Company, Philadelphia.

Russell, A. and Cotton, E. (1994) *The Petö System. Evolution in Britain*, Acorn Press, London.

Scott, S., Caird, F.L. and Williams, B.O. (1985) *Communication in Parkinson's Disease*, Croom Helm, London.

Senelick, R. and Ryan, C. (1991) *Living with Head Injury*, Rehab Hospital Services Corporation.

Shumway-Cook, A. and Woollacott, M. (1995) *Motor control. Theory and Practical Applications*, Williams & Williams, Baltimore.

Simons, A. and Aart, F. (eds) (1984) *Multiple Scelerosis: psychological and social aspects*, Heinemann, London.

Skidmore, D. (1994) *The Ideology of Community Care*, Chapman & Hall, London.

Stanley, R. (1988) Conducive to Change. *Nursing Times*, November 9, vol. 84, No. 45.

Stanton, M. (1992) *Cerebral Palsy. A Practical Guide*, Optima, London.

Stern, G. and Lees, A. (1982) *Parkinson's Disease. The facts*, Oxford University Press.

Sutton, A. (1982) *L.S. Vygotskii on Parkinsonism*. Translation of Volume 1 of L.S. Vygotskii's Complete Works, pp. 109–31.

Sutton, A. (1984) A visit to a class for Parkinson's disease sufferers. Unpublished paper held at National Library for Conductive Education, Birmingham.

Thompson, G.H., Rubin I.L. and Bilenker, R.M. (1983) *Comprehensive Management of Cerebral Palsy*, Grune & Stratton, New York.

Todes, C. (1990) *Shadow Over My Brain. A battle against Parkinson's disease*, The Windrush Press, Gloucestershire.

Tossell, D. and Webb, R. (1994) *Inside the Caring Services, 2nd edn*, Edward Arnold, London.

Twigg, J. and Atkin, K. (1994) *Carers Perceived. Policy and Practice in Informal Care*, Open University Press, Buckingham.

Warlow, C. (ed.) (1987) *Strokes*, MTP Press Limited, Lancaster, England.

Wood, R.L.L. and Eames, P. (eds) (1989) *Models of Brain Injury Rehabilitation*, Chapman & Hall, London.

Youngson, R.M. (1987) *Stroke! A self-help manual for stroke sufferers and their relatives*, BPCC Wheatons Ltd, Exeter.

Useful addresses

Action for Dysphasic Adults (ADA)
1 Royal Street, London. SE1 7LL
Tel: 0171 261 9572
Fax: 0171 928 9542

AFASIC (Overcoming Speech Impairments)
347 Central Markets, Smithfield, London. EC1A 9NH
Tel: 0171 236 3632/6487
Fax: 0171 236 8115

Association of Disabled Professionals
170 Benton Hill, Wakefield Road, Horbury, West Yorkshire. W6 8RF
Tel: 01924 270335
Fax: 01924 276498

Ataxia
Copse Edge, Thursley Road, Elstead, Godalming, Surrey. GU8 6DJ
Tel: 01252 702864
Fax: 01252 703715

British Dyslexia Association
98 London Road, Reading, Berkshire. RG1 5AU
Tel: 01734 662677
Fax: 01734 351927
Helpline: 01734 668271

Carers National Association
20–25 Glasshouse Yard, London. EC1A 4JS
Tel: 0171 490 8818
Fax: 0171 490 8824
Carers Line: 0171 490 8898

Continence Foundation
2 Doughty Street, London. WC1N 2PH
Tel: 0171 404 6875
Fax: 0171 404 6876
Helpline: 0191 213 0050

Disabled Living Foundation
380–4 Harrow Road, London. W9 2HU
Tel: 0171 289 6111
Fax: 0171 266 2922

Dystonia Society
Weddel House, 13–14 West Smithfield, London. EC1A 9HY
Tel: 0171 329 0797
Fax: 0171 329 0689

Headway National Head Injuries Association
7 King Edward Court, King Edward Street, Nottingham. NG1 1EW
Tel: 0115 924 0800
Fax: 0115 924 0432

International Petö Association (for professionals)
Budapest, Kútvölgyi út 6, H-1125, Hungary.
Tel: (361) 201 4533
Fax: (361) 155 6649

MS Under Pressure
(Susie Cornell)
P.O. Box 1270, Chelmsford, Essex. CM2 6BQ
Tel: 01245 252280
Fax: 01245 268098

Multiple Sclerosis Society
25 Effie Road, Fulham, London. SW6 1EE
Tel: 0171 610 7171
Fax: 0171 736 9861
Helpline: 0171 371 8000

Multiple Sclerosis Training, Education and Research Trust
(MUSTER)
P.O. Box 122, Berkhamstead, Herts. HP4 3HA
Fax: 01442 870792

Parkinson's Disease Society
22 Upper Woburn Place, London. WC1H 0RA
Tel: 0171 383 3513
Fax: 0171 383 5754

Petö András Institute
Budapest, Kútvölgyi út 6, H- 1125, Hungary.
Tel: (361) 201 4533
Fax: (361) 155 6649

SCOPE
12 Park Crescent, London. W1N 4EQ
Tel: 0171 636 5020
Fax: 0171 436 2601
Helpline: 0800 626216

Stroke Association
CHSA House, Whitecross Street, London. EC1Y 8JJ
Tel: 0171 490 7999
Fax: 0171 490 2686

The National Institute of Conductive Education
(incorporating National Library of Conductive Education)
Cannon Hill House, Russell Road, Moseley, Birmingham. B13 8RD
Tel: 0121 449 1569
Fax: 0121 449 1611

The UK Federation for Conductive Education
c/o The Hornsey Centre, 26A Dukes Avenue, Muswell Hill, London. N1O
2PT
Tel: 0181 444 7242
Fax: 0181 444 7241

YAPP&RS
c/o Emma Bennion
Warburgh Cottage, Stiffrey, Wells next the Sea, Norfolk. NR33 1QH
Tel: 01485 578603

Index

Page references in **bold** indicate complete chapters. Page numbers in *italic* refer to illustrations.